GOD & YOU CURING CANCER NATURALLY

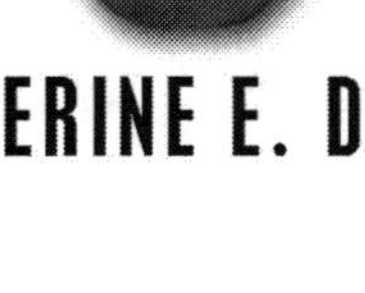

BY KATHERINE E. DELAROSA

The health information expressed in this book is based solely on the personal experience of the author and is not intended as a medical manual. The information should not be used for diagnosis or treatment, or as a substitute for professional medical care. The author and publisher urge you to consult with your health care provider prior to attempting any treatment on yourself or another individual.

God & You, Curing Cancer Naturally.
by Katherine DeLaRosa

God & You, Curing Cancer Naturally.
Published by Katherine DeLaRosa

Contact author: kdelarosa@clcm.net

Printed in the United States of America

ISBN: 978-0-578-11177-3

All scripture quotations taken from the King James Version of the Holy Bible.

ACKNOWLEDGEMENTS

I would like to give thanks to three special people who supported me in the making of this book. Donna Hogue, Nancy Hunt and Regina Lopez for their interest and willingness to share their expertise in proofreading and editing skills. Their combined efforts helped me to complete this book. Thank you very much.

Dedication

To my incredible husband, Manny, who shared with me every step of this journey, I love you. Holding both my hand and my heart he prayed for wisdom as together we sought for answers. To my beautiful and energetic children: Brittany, Jonathon and Timothy, I am grateful for your hugs, words of affirmation, and prayers that brought me through my illness. Next, to my sister, Sandy for your loving sacrifice, you gave beyond measure. To Pastor Nathaniel and Kim Haney for your prayers, advice and spiritual guidance, greatly strengthening my faith. To each of you, I am thankful for your love and compassion. Most of all, to my Lord Jesus Christ for loving me, never leaving me, and leading me to a place of healing.

FORWARD

Very few things have the power to urge a dramatically disciplined change of lifestyle within a matter of months ... but I guess being told you will not live to see your next birthday due to the cancer that has spread throughout your body is one of them.

It was just another normal day at the church office, when the call came through to Kathy that the tiny lump they found was cancerous. Kathy's office is next door to mine and the dark cloud that hovered over us all that day was indescribable. What made it harder was that it was not the first cloud that had appeared that season. We had just lost three precious women of God to this vicious, deadly monster only months and weeks earlier. Would Kathy be another casualty? The battle between faith versus fear began to raise its ugly head as fear seemed to laugh through every negative doctor's report.

I watched Kathy take giant steps of faith as she declared to everyone around her that the Word of God would come to pass in her life through divine healing. I also observed the days when fear seemed to rise up and boldly challenge her faith as the battle of emotions raged inside her mind.

Sunday mornings during worship I watched how Kathy worshiped and praised God with all her heart – even when she was so sick she could hardly stand. The Word of God became her LIFE. It was not just a book that was cracked open on Sunday mornings when the preacher read his Scripture text, but God's promises became Kathy's breath and life. The Word became personal and real to her as God began to "keep her in perfect peace because her mind was stayed on Him" (Isaiah 26:3)

Kathy also began to put legs to her prayers for healing. She was determined to encourage her healing through natural approaches, but did not really know where to start. She prayed for God to guide her as she researched extensively on fighting back through the natural forces God has given to man.

Then it happened one Sunday morning during worship. The presence of God gently swept over and through Kathy's body as His divine healing began to flow. This is her story, and I want her to tell it. What makes this book different is the fact Kathy knows it was the power of God that healed her body that day. This is not some book on health with God sandwiched through it now and then ... this book is about faith, trust and the power of the Word. This book is written by one who believes in divine healing for others who believe in divine healing.

The first part of Kathy's book is a diagnosis. The last part is a prescription. The last part can be applied to all of our lives whether we have battled with a terminal disease or not. May the nuggets of gold that were given to Kathy through this battle be passed down to each reader in hopes of renewing us in body, soul, and spirit.

Kim Haney,
Pastor of Women's Ministries
Christian Life Center
Stockton, California

CONTENTS

Introduction

The past two years brought unprecedented change in my life. God saw fit to allow a crisis to enter my life and that of my family. Nothing in my past adequately prepared me for the impact this change would bring.

On October 5, 2010, I was diagnosed with breast cancer. Almost overnight, I found myself waging a personal war against a very misunderstood and terrifying enemy. The very mention of the word "cancer" brought feelings of despair. Without question, I was lost and fearful in the place of incurable diseases. Surrounded by this unseen enemy, I heard the boasting of past victories from inside the secure world of a modern healthcare system.

Within this system, I found few answers and little hope for my future. Somehow, I knew I was far off course, headed for certain destruction. In desperation, I prayed for a way out. Believing God was the source of my help, I reached out to embrace His loving touch. He alone became my guide, unfolding a map and revealing to me the path I should choose. Together, we charted a course that would ultimately lead to a place of healing. Along the way, I found shelter in the knowledge of this singular truth: ...*With men it is impossible, but not with God: for with God all things are possible.* (Mark 10:27)

Within the pages of this book, I offer encouragement and hope that God will remove your fear and empower you to connect with the source of your healing. Along with spiritual insights, I have included practical and technical information to give you a clear understanding of the natural process behind preventing and curing cancer. God is faithful to His Word. He will provide the courage and the answers necessary for you to safely arrive at your destination of healing.

part one

My Story

The year started out with great promise. Our daughter, Brittany, was a senior in high school, and we looked forward to her graduation. It seemed as though my husband, Manny, and I spent months making preparations for the celebration, all the while reminiscing over how quickly eighteen years had disappeared. Still, all the planning was fun, even in the midst of our very busy schedules. We both worked full-time and were very involved with our church. My husband's job as an executive kept him ever pushing for higher ground, as well as juggling a very demanding travel schedule. In fact, his travel that year would take him once again to Germany. As a bonus, Manny decided to take Brittany to Germany as her graduation present. In between work and travel, we managed school and sports for our twin boys. Jonathon and Timothy were always on the move, playing baseball, flag football and basketball. We were like so many other families with plenty of activities packed into our daily schedule.

After our daughter's graduation, the hot summer months stretched out before us. Summer is, without a doubt, my favorite time of year. We now live in Stockton, California, as our family made the long journey here from Florida after Manny accepted a job promotion. For us, living in California meant being far away from our family. To help bridge the distance, we always tried to plan at least one vacation every year by returning to Florida. That year we had the fortunate circumstances of planning a vacation around an already scheduled business retreat to Fort Lauderdale with Manny's job. His job would make it possible for us to extend our time in Florida and visit

Manny's family in Miami. As it was, his father was coping with lung cancer, and we needed to spend time with him.

Going through chemotherapy made things difficult for his dad. My sister-in-law was the point person for his care, but she had her own family. This was not the best of circumstances. At any rate, we stayed in touch, giving our support in any way possible. We lifted Manny's dad up in prayer many times, asking God to heal him. At the time, we were as informed as most people were about cancer. We knew the reality of this disease and, like everyone else, believed existing treatments were effective. Certainly, we trusted that his physicians were doing their best to bring him into remission.

Keeping in mind that this was a business trip, we made plans to balance our time between visiting family and enjoying the beautiful beaches. Everyone knew we were coming from California and the thought of reuniting with family made the trip even more exciting. Originally, Manny's family came to Miami from Cuba. Like so many people in south Florida, they escaped after Castro overthrew Batista's government in 1959 and started life over again in Miami.

Cubans are a proud people, holding close to their cultural traditions. I have always admired and enjoyed experiencing this influence that has remained alive in their family for generations. One of my favorite things to look forward to was the incredible Cuban cuisine. In fact, our family began to talk about all of the great food we would enjoy long before we ever left home.

Once we arrived in Fort Lauderdale, Manny made contact with his family and soon learned that his dad had taken a turn for the worst. He had been hospitalized with breathing problems, and the family was greatly concerned. Needless to say, we were surprised to hear the news and quickly changed our plans to get to the hospital. We arrived, making sure that our kids were with us so that they could see their grandfather. Making our way through the hospital floors and long hallways, we finally arrived at his room. I will never forget the image of his lying in a hospital bed. The bed seemed so big compared to his thin, frail body. He managed to raise his arm, waving to us as we entered the door. A smile came across his face, assuring us, of how glad he was that we were there. It was hard to recognize him. He had lost all of his hair, and his face was so pale and thin that he did not look like himself. We were not prepared for this. Brittany broke into tears and hid her face, while the rest of us remained composed. We surrounded Manny's dad and his wife with hugs. I could see the concern and shock on Manny's face. How had this happened? Why didn't we know he was in this condition? All we knew was that he was undergoing treatment, and everyone was hopeful for his recovery.

The following day Manny notified his job. Under the circumstances, he would not be able to attend meetings as scheduled. The next few days turned into a roller coaster ride of emotions. We spent our time at the hospital, visiting with family members and engaging doctors whenever possible. All we wanted to understand was why his health was failing so quickly. Day by day he was getting worse, and it seemed as though decisions made by the doctors did not improve his condition. It was obvious that the hospital did not expect him to recover. All arrangements for his care were out of our hands, as we watched the hospital transfer him to different rooms, resulting in less medical attention each time. Finally, a decision was made to administer morphine. I did not understand much about his battle with lung cancer, but I did know that morphine was a one-way trip. Once he began taking morphine there would be no turning around. Within a few short days we had gone from talking and engaging with his dad to standing next to the bedside of an unconscious man. At one point, I stepped out of the room and asked a nurse how she thought he was doing. She responded that, in her experience, he had only hours to live.

Those next few hours were priceless. Manny continued to speak with his dad, even though he never really was able to respond. The room was filled with family and friends giving each other support. Manny's uncle, Luis, and his wife, Terri, stood close to his bedside. Together we shared our faith that God was able to transcend all of the grief we felt. Terri leaned down and began singing a beautiful, soft, worship song. We all began to pray that God would touch Manny's dad, as well as everyone gathered in the hospital room. God was amazing. His presence was felt in such a strong way. Although Manny's dad never expressed faith in God, we were grateful that God responded. Time stood still as we witnessed his fragile life slip away. The next few days were spent trying to console ourselves, as we relived the experience in unbelief. We had never dealt with a family member facing cancer. There were many unanswered questions about his illness and the care he had received. We were only left with the uneasy feeling that his father's illness should have had a much different outcome.

Our family returned home, saddened by our experience and dreading the daily routine that would beckon us to move past our loss. Those early days quickly turned into weeks, as we said goodbye to the summer months. We certainly love the summer, but we do our best to look forward to the changing of the season and the onset of a new school year. This school year would be different. We made the decision to home school our boys. I had spent the summer months enrolling them in a charter school and getting their curriculum in order. I knew home school would be a challenge, but I was truly looking forward to this new adventure.

As usual, that time of year our mailbox filled up with all of the reminders for dental appointments, eye exams and routine medical exams. I was diligent about making these appointments, especially for my children. However, that particular year, I had already postponed my routine mammogram even before our trip to Florida. I knew the appointment would not take long, but other things kept pushing it forward. Once again, the appointment reminder card was staring me in the face. There were no more excuses. I simply had to get it done, and I knew that I would feel relieved once the mammogram was complete.

A couple of weeks went by, and I received another information card in the mail. It was small and unassuming. I almost didn't open it, because I was certain that it would contain the same routine message informing me of my good test results. After opening the card, I found myself rereading the message several times. It simply stated that the results were abnormal and that I needed to call for a follow-up appointment. My first reaction was annoyance by the inconvenience that this would most certainly cause. After all, there was nothing really wrong. I knew that I was careful with my health, and there were no signs of any concerns.

My husband and I kept the news to ourselves. We did not want to send up any unnecessary alarms. As instructed, I followed up with a call to discuss the results. I was told that the mammogram showed small calcifications in the right breast tissue. These are common but can be a precursor to breast cancer. I did my best to push for more information about these results, but it was obvious that my only avenue was to take the next recommended step of a biopsy. As the conversation continued, the patient advisor explained the simplicity and necessity of the procedure in a positive and encouraging tone. Still not wanting to believe that this could be serious, I agreed to schedule the biopsy, almost as a means to defy any possibility for concern. For some unexplained reason, I did not react as usual to thoroughly question and research such a decision. I could not seem to grasp even the possibility that any test would result in a positive finding. In fact, I played down the situation and reassured Manny that I would be fine.

I had not yet realized the effect that this decision was weighing on me. Every day, I went to work as usual and thought I was concealing everything. I tried not to let on to what I was potentially facing. My husband and I believe in the power of prayer and speaking positively about any situation in our lives. It only seemed natural for us to remain calm and wait for this storm to pass. However, my office manager, Alisha, caught me by surprise one afternoon as she expressed her concern. She told me that she had noticed I was not quite myself and wondered about the time I had requested to be out of the office. I remember hesitating for a moment before telling her exactly what I was facing. I knew that I could count on her to be supportive, and it only seemed fair to be honest. She immediately offered her prayers, as I maintained everything would be all right.

I scheduled a full day for the appointment. Unfortunately, I had to drive some distance to the medical facility where the biopsy was performed. It had been explained to me that this procedure was routine and noninvasive. I had been given the distinct impression there was nothing adverse for me to consider about undergoing this procedure. Clearly, I operated on the belief that having this biopsy was in my best interest. In my mind, this biopsy would simply confirm that the calcifications were benign.

I arrived on schedule, anxious to get this behind me. I quickly checked in and took a seat in the rather large lobby area. A hundred thoughts ran through my mind, as I stared at the other people sitting around me. How many of them were here for a similar procedure? There were both young and old patients, each representing the possibility of something serious. As I scanned the room, I realized how suddenly a health issue could over take one's life. Everything comes to a standstill. All plans are put on hold and nothing matters until you have answers. As I contemplated this, it occurred to me that I had been waiting almost 45 minutes. Immediately, an uneasy feeling came over me, and I wanted to get up and dash out the door. I was nervous and doubtful about going through with the biopsy. My mind began to juggle a list of reasons to stay or to go. In that indecisive moment, I heard my name called. Startled, I pushed all of those negative feelings aside and followed the nurse into the appointment room. I was briefed about the procedure and asked to sign a standard consent form. Then, a technician guided me to another room, where I put on a gown and received more instructions from the doctor. The procedure was awkward and uncomfortable.

It involved the precision targeting of a needle into the breast to extract tissue samples from the areas in question. This was done several times to obtain sufficient samples for the lab. I left feeling unsure about the whole experience, knowing I would most certainly be bruised for days from this procedure.

It took almost a week before the results were available. I was so convinced that everything would be fine that I opted to be notified by phone. The call came while I was still at work in my office. The voice was calm and simply gave me the news that the results were positive for invasive ductal carcinoma. I was also made aware that my breast cancer was HER2-positive. This meant that the cancer tested positive for a protein called human epidermal growth factor 2 (HER2), which promotes the rapid growth of cancer cells. Of course, I wanted as much information as possible. My head was swimming with unanswered questions, as I rapidly fired at least ten of my concerns into the phone. She did her best to give me more facts about my type of breast cancer, but every word was delivered in a cautious manner. I realized she purposely stayed in the middle of the road, remaining neutral with her expressions as she responded. It was obvious that I had reached the end of this phone call. Avoiding a rush of emotions, I kindly thanked her and excused myself from the conversation.

I do not even remember my picking up my phone again, but suddenly Manny was listening to the sound of my shaken voice telling him the bad news. He paused at first and then told me that he was picking up his things and would be on the road headed home. I filled him in on everything that I knew from my phone call, and we spoke only of a positive outcome. We agreed to talk more after we both got home. Later that day, I gathered up my things and excused myself, after telling my office manager the news. She understood that I was in no shape to stay or to share this news with everyone. I just asked her to please let the Pastor know that we needed prayer.

I easily made it home before Manny, as he had a long drive from his office. Once there, I waited patiently, knowing that we did not want to tell our children until he arrived. It made sense for all of us to be together to hopefully help them cope. When I heard Manny's car pull in the driveway, I quickly went out to meet him. We embraced and I felt safe once again. As we separated, he looked at me and said that he had called my sister. Manny knew that I had chosen to keep the news between us. I wanted to believe this would pass without a need to worry anyone. The thought of my sister knowing brought me to tears. It was simply the final straw in keeping back the emotions that had piled up until that moment. I had resisted Manny's decision to call anyone, but at this point, it was the right thing to do. After I collected myself, we both went into the house and called our children together. We did our best to soften the news and deliver it in a way that would not frighten them. However, Brittany was old enough to know the serious implications of my diagnosis, and we knew they would all think about the recent loss of their grandfather. With this in mind, Manny pulled us all together in a tight circle and prayed that God would heal my body and strengthen all of us during this difficult time.

The following morning we were all up as usual, moving through our morning routine. It was helpful to know that life would not come to a standstill. After all, we both had jobs to fulfill, plus school and everyday activities for our family. Our kids needed to know that we were going to be okay. In light of this, I was determined to keep our schedule normal in every way possible. That day would be no different. After getting dressed, I made my way upstairs to our family room. Each morning we set aside time to read our Bibles together. For most of that year, we had been in the Old Testament, and on that particular morning we were on chapter 38 of the book of Isaiah. I began reading slowly, making sure they listened and understood. I had read only a few verses when the story struck at the heart of my situation. The prophet Isaiah was sent by God unto King Hezekiah to deliver very sobering news. God revealed to King Hezekiah that the time had come for him to die. He was very sick, and the word from God was clear; King Hezekiah would not recover. Upon reading this, I felt fear grip me. I tried not to show any hesitation in my voice, but I could not help thinking, "Was this story speaking directly of my future?"

Immediately upon receiving the news, King Hezekiah responded by turning his face and crying out to God. He reminded God that he had been a righteous king before Israel and so he asked God to spare his life. His prayer was one of a desperate man not ashamed of his tears, as he humbled himself and asked God to heal him. Ultimately, he prayed a powerful prayer, and it moved the heart of God to grant him fifteen more years. At the point of reading this, I was convinced God was indeed speaking to me. There simply was no coincidence in having read that particular passage of Scripture the day after my diagnosis. I felt the chapter was a road map or a set of instructions. The more I read, the more I began to understand God's desire to heal me. The loving relationship between God and King Hezekiah was the key in this passage.

"Behold, for peace I had great bitterness: but thou has in love to my soul delivered it from the pit of corruption: for thou hast cast all my sins behind thy back" (Isaiah 38:17).

It was clear to me that God felt Hezekiah's sorrow and responded out of a great love for the King. It is also true that King Hezekiah loved God. He was grateful that his life had been spared and returned praise and love to the One who had saved him.

For the grave cannot praise thee, death can not celebrate thee: they that go down into the pit cannot hope for thy truth. The living, the living, he shall praise thee, as I do this day: the father to the children shall make known thy truth. The Lord was ready to save me: therefore we will sing my songs to the stringed instruments all the days of our life in the house of the Lord. Isaiah 38:18-20

I continued reading through the end of the chapter where the prophet Isaiah instructed King Hezekiah to make a paste of figs and use it as a healing salve. At the time, I did not know those verses would prove to mirror my own path to healing.

Over the next week, I determined to continue to search the Bible for every Scripture on the topic of healing. I wanted to know everything about how and why God healed someone. I marveled as I read through the gospels at the miraculous healings that took place. Two things stood out to me in all of my reading. First, Jesus had great compassion on those who were sick. Second, people believed that Jesus had the power to heal them. An expression of faith was evident in every healing. How simple and yet how profound this concept is. Little by little, I was moving toward my answer. God gently spoke to me in time of prayer, through reading His words and through the people He placed in my life.

The next few days blended together, as I anxiously waited for my consultation with a surgeon. During that time, I searched online for information that related to breast cancer. I wanted to be informed before any decisions were made regarding surgery. I also bought several books on the subject, hoping to better understand my options. At the appointment, Manny and I listened carefully as the surgeon reviewed images from the pathology report. By all indications, the cancer was contained in a microscopic area of tissue. This was good news because the cancer had obviously been detected early. The recommended procedure for my case would be a routine lumpectomy.

During that same week, I began exploring options for alternative medicine. I had been on the phone constantly with Sandy, sharing updates and information. She did research on her end, using her own resources. Through her encouragement, I began eating exclusively organic and included certain supplements in my diet. At the same time, my pastor and his wife, Nathaniel and Kim Haney, were a great support to me both spiritually and in my search for safer treatments. Kim Haney gave me a referral to a holistic doctor in our area. She provided further insight into the healing possibilities of natural medicines.

My surgery date was scheduled in two weeks. I planned to use the time seeking every safe option available, including the surgical procedure. My surgeon had not yet discussed any possibility of radiation treatments following surgery. However, I knew from my research that was often the case. I shared my concern with Manny, as we both were working to find answers. Almost immediately he realized that the company he worked for manufactured a medical device called Intraoperative Radiation Therapy, (IORT). Through it radiation could be administered during surgery. The radiation would be delivered precisely and only to the surgery site. This is a much preferable option to radiating the entire breast. With this information, I began petitioning my surgeon and insurance company to allow this procedure, in the event radiation was necessary. I also searched for any clinical trials that might provide a better outcome from surgery. Needless to say, we were doing our best to be proactive so that, hopefully, I would not look back with any regrets post surgery.

By that time, a week had passed since I received my biopsy results. In an effort to gain more information and to insure that I had a true picture of my condition, I made an appointment to see a surgeon for a second opinion. I purposely chose a female surgeon, believing that her perspective would be encouraging, or at least sympathetic, to all of my concerns. Up until that point, I had felt isolated and uninformed in a medical system that did not see me as an individual but as an insurance number on a small plastic card. While I did not quite understand it, the healthcare system saw me as only one of countless women who would face that same crisis. Ironically, my diagnosis had come in the month of October: the month set aside for breast cancer awareness. Everywhere I went I saw pink ribbons and balloons and yet, for all this "awareness" as a patient, I was not very aware of my options. With that mind set, I was anxious to get a second opinion. Perhaps the next surgeon would have better insight or see the test results in a different light.

Two days before my appointment, I began to notice a change in my breast. The area around the biopsy site was swollen and felt harder than the surrounding tissue. I told Manny, and we agreed this would be a priority when I met with the surgeon. I tried not to be alarmed, but it weighed heavily on my mind. Any change at this point was a signal to me that something was wrong. By the next evening I decided to call the patient help line to speak with a nurse. Unfortunately, the nurse would not comment on the change in my breast. I would have to wait until the following morning to see the surgeon. At the doctor's office, I went through the routine check in procedure before changing into a gown. It did not take long before I heard a knock at the door, and the doctor entered the small examination room. She sat down, politely introduced herself, and reassured me she had reviewed my biopsy report. She paused and smiled before leaning forward, indicating it was now my turn to speak. Without hesitation, I began with a list of questions and concerns, including a reality check on the validity of the report. Sadly, she confirmed the diagnosis and agreed with the recommendation for a lumpectomy. I felt her answers came too quickly, as if they had been "copied and pasted" into a document. I had the sinking feeling that no matter how many doctors I spoke with, the outcome would be the same. I decided to shift the conversation to the pressing concern of the recent change I had experienced. Lying down, she began the examination while asking basic questions about when the biopsy was done and when I took off the bandages, etc. Finally, she concluded that the tissue had been bruised during the procedure. Explaining to me how the needle punctures the tissue multiple times often causing soreness and swelling. It all sounded plausible, but for some reason I did not feel relieved as expected.

Over the next few days I continued my normal schedule, remaining prayerful about the upcoming surgery. Each day at work my coworkers offered words of encouragement. I admit it was not easy to receive the attention my illness had brought. Manny and I had always been on the other side, giving to someone else in a time of need. However, there was great comfort in every sincere and positive word I heard. Nothing could replace a smile, a hug or just a look, expressing love and concern. Most importantly, we had the support of everyone's prayers. I remember a comment my coworker, Vickie, made to me after we prayed together. She told me that God would bring me through my illness and use my experience to bless others. God was truly amazing in the unexpected people He placed in my path.

I remember specifically meeting an instructor for lunch to discuss home schooling for my sons. I had not had the opportunity to share with her what had happened with my diagnosis. However, as our lunch meeting was winding down, she casually asked me how things were going. I took that moment to update her on what had transpired over the past week and a half. Although she was sympathetic, the news did not seem to alarm her. Instead, she began to tell me the story of her own son's battle with cancer. As an infant, he had been diagnosed with stage IV, neuroblastoma carcinoma. He was considered a high-risk patient that was unlikely to respond to treatments. Immediately, her family reacted by reaching out to everyone asking for prayer. Her husband even called local churches requesting to be placed on prayer lists. She testified about their faith and how God miraculously healed their son. She ended her story by adding they had been placed in a study of ten families with children who had this same type of cancer. Out of the ten families their son was the only one who survived. I thanked her for sharing her story, as it had greatly strengthened me. As I drove away from the restaurant, I remembered thinking if God could heal her son of stage IV cancer, then he could certainly heal me.

The following day I had an appointment to discuss the Intraoperative Radiation Therapy procedure that I had requested for my surgery. At this appointment the doctor reviewed my report and then proceeded with an examination. She flinched as she opened up my gown and, with a very stern face, commented on how large the tumor was. Quickly, I corrected her by telling her that the firmness in my breast was due to bruising from the biopsy. I continued to fill her in on my recent appointments, carefully providing all of the details. Unresponsive to me, she backed up from the examination table and quickly picked up the phone. Her voice urgently requested to speak with my doctor, who was scheduled to perform the surgery. Upon hanging up the phone, she told me to get dressed and immediately go to his office. The urgency in her voice made me nervous as she refused any further discussion about the procedure. In a matter of minutes I reached the surgeon's office. My heart was pounding as I fumbled in my purse for my insurance card. Next, the receptionist called for a nurse, and I was quickly ushered into a room where the surgeon waited to see me. After examining me once again, he told me that he had to consider something else was causing those changes. True enough, the swelling and firmness had greatly increased, and he indicated this was more than mere bruising of the tissue. Continuing, he explained this might be a large blood clot resulting from the biopsy. Furthermore, if it was a large blood clot nothing could be done except to remove the entire breast. I sat there frozen in disbelief. How casually he had made that statement without regard for what this news would mean to me. Before anything could be determined I would have to undergo yet another mammogram.

While walking to the radiology department I quickly phoned Manny. I was barely able to speak, as my voice was choked with tears. He managed to calm me down by reminding me that nothing had been decided, and it would do me no good to be so upset at this point. He assured me he would be on the road, heading my way soon. As I waited in the lobby of the radiology department, I glanced up to see Alisha walking toward me. Manny had called her to come and be with me, as he was at least an hour's drive from the medical office. She gave me a hug, sat down next to me and listened, as I explained what had just happened. Finally, a technician called my name and ushered me back for the screening. The process did not take long and the digital file was immediately available for my doctor. We sat together in his office reviewing the results. Unfortunately, he indicated the image was not clear enough to make a determination. Instead, I would have to return the following morning for a sonogram.

Once again, Manny and I sat holding hands anxiously awaiting my appointment. It was early in the morning, a little after 7:00 a.m. We were scheduled early, due to a full booking in the department. The radiologist and technician had both agreed to come in early, just to accommodate my sonogram. The lobby area was quite large, and it seemed ominous without the usual noise and constant flow of people. I stared at the double doors leading into the department; slowly they opened, and a nurse walked briskly out, smiling as she approached us. She directed us to the examination room where I was prepped for the procedure. Within minutes the technician entered the room and casually engaged both of us, as if to try and relieve the obvious tension we were feeling. There was simply no way I could hide my anxiety. By now I was tired of the whole examination process, and it showed. Manny smiled at me with a reassuring look, doing his best to help me with the situation. While explaining our dilemma, the technician preformed the sonogram. We cautiously asked questions, hoping to gain insight into what the sonogram might reveal. However, her response was clear. The radiologist was the only one that could discuss the results. Realizing our need for answers, she quickly left the room, calling for the radiologist. Moments later the radiologist entered the room, sat down and promptly told us he had seen the images in his office, and there was no evidence of a large blood clot. Before we could react to this bit of good news, he hit us hard by telling us it appeared to be a case of inflammatory breast cancer. He advised us to immediately return to my surgeon's office for a consultation, and then he exited the room as quickly as he had entered. We were devastated, and I felt a sickening feeling come over me. In searching for information about my own breast cancer, I had become aware of this very rare and aggressive form of cancer.

After getting dressed, I collected my belongings, and we made our way back to the surgery department to see my doctor. While reviewing the sonogram, he made no reference to the possibility of inflammatory breast cancer. Instead, he refrained from such comments. He told us the standard procedure, in this case, would be another biopsy. There was simply no way to know what was causing the changes without having a pathology report from a new tissue sample. As my doctor put it, he could not move forward without the report. I found myself in a no-win situation. I had already seen enough evidence supporting the idea that a biopsy causes cancer to spread. With our backs against the wall I made the only possible decision, to proceed with the procedure. My only request was that the sample be expedited to the lab in light of my pressing circumstances.

Over the next couple of days, I turned my focus back on searching for more understanding about healing, as well as natural medicine. I found great comfort in reading every possible Scripture that related to healing. It was amazing how many passages throughout the Bible touch on this subject. Some were specific stories about physical healing, while others spoke of emotional and spiritual healing. Regardless of the emphasis, I made every verse my own promise.

One afternoon I was on the phone with Sandy talking about what I was reading, and she told me of several encouraging books she had read on the subject. Ironically, she was also dealing with her own need for healing from a kidney disease. During this time, we formed our own small support group, praying for each other and sharing our research and experiences. She was already on a path to pursue natural medicine. In fact, I was thankful for her advise to change my diet to organic foods and to include essential supplements in my healthcare regimen. She continued to tell me about a woman who had inoperable cancer. The doctors had given her only a few weeks to live. As a woman of faith, she turned to God. Believing her answer was in the Bible, she began to read and collect favorite Scriptures on healing. Every day she purposed to read and pray over those same Scriptures. In fact, she described her time of reading as if she were taking medicine, reading and rereading verses until most of them were committed to memory. Weeks turned into months and then months into years. Without explanation, her doctor pronounced her free of cancer. For her, the answer was obvious; she had been healed by the power of God's Word.

It had been nearly two weeks since my diagnosis, and we were a bit anxious to get the latest results from the biopsy. Needless to say, I had made several calls to the doctor's office, thinking the results would be available – only to be disappointed. By now it was apparent my test results would take a full week to process. As I drove home from work, I realized I was juggling so many thoughts about what I was facing. It was difficult just trying to understand the impact of all of this and the decisions that still lay ahead. My future was uncertain, and for the first time in my life, I could not figure this out nor could I control the situation. Even in this turmoil, I felt God urging me to turn my thoughts toward Him. It was only in those moments that I could truly feel the peace I so desperately needed. By the time I arrived home, I had put any disappointments from the day behind me. It was time to enjoy my family and catch up on their busy day.

Later in the evening, I headed to my bedroom to shower and get ready for the night. I stood in the shower longer than usual, hoping the hot water would relax my tired neck muscles. Looking down, I saw what appeared to be swelling in mid-center of my chest. The lighting was not really good, so I thought, perhaps, I was really not seeing it clearly. Turning off the water, I stepped out and stood directly underneath the bathroom light. There was no mistake; the swelling was quite obvious now. Calling out to Manny, I wrapped myself in a towel and walked out into our bedroom. As he entered the room, I pointed to my chest, and he acknowledged my same observation.

Watching him shake his head, I simply could not speak. We both were thinking the same thing. The cancer was growing out of control. It had engulfed my right breast and was now crossing over the center chest area.

I glanced at the clock by our bed; it was now 8:00 p.m. There was no way I was going to wait until the next morning. The cancer had already taken full advantage of the time waiting for the biopsy results. All I could think of was that we needed to act now. Grabbing my phone, I rushed through the voicemail prompts trying to get through to the medical call center. Finally, a nurse was available, and I shared my circumstances asking for a call back from my surgeon. She politely gave me the standard response, instructing me to call during regular office hours. To this I forcefully responded that I believed my life was threatened. Upon hearing these words she agreed to contact my surgeon immediately. At the same time, Manny called Sandy to make flight arrangements for her to arrive the next day. While we waited for my surgeon to call, I also phoned Alisha, updating her on what was happening. She offered to have the executive associate pastor, Eli Lopez, call Manny. For us, this was an emergency, and we wanted all the prayer support possible. It took only minutes before we were both on separate phone calls, trying to sort out our next move. Reluctantly, I knew surgery was the only conceivable option. By the time my call ended, we had agreed to meet the surgeon at a hospital in a neighboring city.

Once again, our family stood together holding hands in a tight circle as Manny prayed. The hardest thing I did was to look into the faces of my children, knowing they would have to stay alone at the house. Unfortunately, it was already late, and we had no idea what the next day would bring. With a concerned look, Brittany reassured us she would have no trouble taking care of her twin brothers. We said our goodbyes, promising to check in with them often. As we drove off, I looked back again, repeating a prayer for God to watch over them.

We arrived at the hospital, making quick time of the check-in process.

Looking around, only a few people could be seen in the entire building. Due to the late hour, my surgeon had received special permission to assemble a surgical team. Although I understood the procedure, we were briefed in detail, finally giving our permission to proceed with a modified radical mastectomy and axillary node dissection. Simultaneously, I was prepped for surgery and, in no time, was on my way to the operating room. Manny disappeared down the hall and into a lobby area, where his close friend Tom was waiting. By 1:00 a.m. the surgery was over, and I was wheeled back into recovery. I remember waking up trying to adjust to the tight bandages around my chest – feeling no pain except for the knowledge of what a surgeon's scalpel had just accomplished.

Mid-morning brought a flurry of activity to my room, including a nurse checking my vital signs. She was overly friendly, offering comforting words and reminding me that plenty of women face this same surgery. Continuing on, she rattled off a list of every available plastic surgeon, should I choose to undergo reconstructive surgery in the future. Manny and I both managed to smile and thank her for being so positive and informative. Next, we were surprised to hear that everything checked out fine, and my surgeon had already signed release forms. This was the best news all morning. Admittedly, recovering at home was preferable to staying in a hospital bed. Without hesitation, I accepted help getting dressed, and the wheelchair ride out to the hospital entrance where Manny waited with our car.

The drive home gave us a chance to soak in the moments together and be grateful for being on the other side of surgery. Arriving home, we were greeted with smiles and a rush of hugs. God had answered our prayers to bring us all together again. Wasting no time, Manny spun around and headed back out the door to pick up Sandy at the airport. By now, I was resting comfortably in one of our living room chairs with my kids gathered around, asking endless questions about my hospital stay and filling me in on their adventures at home without us. When things settled down, Brittany told me how she had laid on her bedroom floor praying throughout the night. In that moment, I understood for the first time the value of knowing someone else was praying. We continued talking until Manny arrived back home with Sandy from the airport. With a brave face, Sandy hugged me, and we both agreed how good it was to be together.

Over the next few days, friends and church family visited our home. Bringing a different level of comfort and sharing their faith for a complete recovery. We were blessed to receive meals prepared by caring hands and a host of cards, phone calls and beautiful flowers. In fact, we were simply overwhelmed with the outpouring of support. In between the well wishes and prayers, came the harsh reality of waiting on a pathology report that left us facing an uncertain future.

Once situated, Sandy and Manny began executing their own plans to turn our home into a haven for healing. They discussed everything, from new sources for healthy foods and products to reorganizing our kitchen to accommodate a natural healing approach to preparing foods. One of the first things that changed was our drinking water. Manny ordered and installed a reverse osmosis water filtration system under our kitchen sink. This allowed for a pure source of water for both drinking and cooking. Sandy brought a love for cooking with her, and together with Brittany, they prepared new and nutritious foods for me throughout the day. In every moment of the day, Sandy searched online for a better understanding of the role natural medicine played in the healing process. Sharing her enthusiasm with me, I was beginning to see the possibilities of my own role in reclaiming my health.

A few days later the phone call finally came with news of my test results. With a steady voice, my surgeon carefully explained he had removed 10 lymph nodes from under my right arm with all but one expressing positive for cancer. Upon hearing this news, I immediately knew I was now dealing with stage III cancer. Soon I would receive a call to schedule a follow-up visit with an oncologist. It now seemed as if everything happened much too quickly. I found myself caught up in the inertia of events well out of my control. The "system" was moving me methodically through a carefully-planned patient process. Manny broke the awkward silence by reminding me that God was in control, and Sandy joined in by adding He would bless my efforts in turning around this crisis.

Before long, Manny and I found ourselves sitting in another waiting area at the medical center. We were here for my first consultation with an oncologist. I had spent several days combing the Internet, compiling information on stage III breast cancer. From my research, I had typed up a list of questions regarding possible treatment options. My hope was to be prepared enough to stay focused and not miss any details affecting future decisions. Once in the examination room, we sat next to each other with our eyes scanning the room. A poster caught our attention. It advertised Herceptin, a fairly new cancer drug designed to block aggressive growth receptors associated with my HER2-positive diagnosis. It also displayed some very grave survival statistics, even with the effectiveness of this new medication. Manny looked at me and gently squeezed my hand. Before he could speak, the doctor entered the room. She was polite enough but very stern, reviewing the pathology report and confirming my stage III status. Referring to my condition, she emphasized the word "serious." Then she moved right into the next phase of scheduling a series of diagnostic tests. As she talked, I tried hard to study her face and movements, looking for any sign that would communicate something positive. However, her words were well rehearsed, almost scripted. It seemed as if she had purposely learned to deal with her patients, void of emotion. Perhaps this type of investment had proven to be too costly. Finally, she unfolded her recommendation for six rounds of two chemotherapy drugs, accompanied by Herceptin. My treatment would begin promptly after the diagnostic screening was complete and continue over a six-month time frame.

Chemotherapy, was a word I dreaded hearing. Knowing this would be the only option presented, I had spent considerable time reading about these different types of cancer drugs. It really did not matter which drug I researched, the side effects seemed across the board detrimental to the over-all goal of healing. I was also aware of their poor track record for sustainable results in cancer patients. I found myself in a race against time, searching for answers that would possibly provide an alternative to traditional medicine. At this point, I had learned just enough; convincing me that a solution, indeed, existed.

I spent the next couple of weeks enduring a series of diagnostic imaging. Manny and I traveled to different hospitals, accommodating various tests. Those tests included a CT scan, MRI, and a bone scan. Although I was hesitant to undergo repeated exposure to radiation, my doctor convinced me there was no other way to have a complete understanding of my condition. As the days passed, I found myself increasingly consumed with everything associated to my illness. My days were scheduled around appointments and lab results. In between, questions and research prioritized the agenda of each day. Even though my world had turned upside down, Manny and I trusted God. I was also very blessed to have Sandy adding her encouragement. We could talk for hours, reminiscing on the many times God had answered prayers throughout our lives. We both drew strength from these moments, counting on the faithfulness of our God.

By now it was late October and there was only one thing on all our minds. We were waiting for any word on the results of my imaging scans. It was early afternoon when the call came. Sandy and I had finished our lunch and were engaged in conversation when the phone rang. I recognized my doctor's voice and immediately knew why she had called. Bracing myself, she told me she had received the results from my CT and MRI scans. Both scans confirmed the cancer had spread to my liver, lymph nodes in the center chest area and possibly a vertebra in my back. She finished by telling me I needed to begin chemotherapy as soon as possible. As I put the phone down and looked at Sandy, tears filled my eyes. With this news, my condition had escalated to stage IV cancer. We sat together in silence for a few moments, just trying to take in the news. I really could not speak, as emotions held my voice captive. This feeling was intensified by seeing one of my children pass through the dining room unaware of the call I had received. A hundred thoughts ran through my mind, but none so gripping as the thought of not being here for my children.

I had strongly resisted the idea of chemotherapy. Manny and I had discussed all of the adverse issues surrounding this treatment. However, I needed more time to formulate an alternative treatment plan. We had been doing our homework, but I only had bits and pieces of a workable plan. My cancer had grown at such a rapid pace that not even the doctors could explain what had happened. There was no way of knowing how fast the cancer would continue to spread. At this point, I found myself needing advice and direction. I trusted Manny to give me every chance possible to follow after alternative medicine, but he could not help being swayed by the current change of events. Both Manny and Sandy now believed chemotherapy might be the only sure way to slow down the cancer, providing me the time I needed to secure a safer path to healing.

Lying in bed each night, I entered into a solitary place. Retreating from the day, I was able to remove myself from the pressures weighing on me and simply share my hurts and fears with God. I told Him everything that concerned me. Even now it is hard to describe the overwhelming comfort I felt in the face of increasingly bad news. Many times I spent the night just thanking God for giving me one more day. I thanked Him for letting me feel Manny's love and to embrace each of my children. Nothing was taken for granted. Beyond this, I had learned to meditate on specific Bible verses, allowing them to drowned out the negative voices surrounding me. God's love was inescapably building a stronger faith within me.

Finally, I agreed to my oncologist's recommendation for chemotherapy.

I admit there was some relief, just knowing the decision was over. In order to expedite things, I requested to forgo the usual orientation process choosing rather to jump into the preliminary consultation and necessary lab work. This also included a decision to acquire a chest port. I was aware of the damage chemotherapy would cause my veins. A chest port was the only way I could protect against this certainty. After the necessary blood work was complete, the day of my first treatment arrived. Unbeknownst to me, I was about to enter the secret sanctum of the infusion center. This department was a series of well-connected, secured rooms within the medical facility. After being checked in and receiving my ID bracelet, Manny and I were taken into one of the treatment areas where my oncology nurse greeted us. We were taken to an individual treatment area fully equipped for the infusion process. The nursing station was in the center of the room surrounded by individual infusion chairs covering every available inch of wall space.

The oncology nurse began the methodical process of preparing for infusion. Before chemotherapy, I would have to take several IV solutions including Beneydryl® to prevent an allergic reaction. This entire process took several hours to complete. In between these infusions, Manny and I took full notice of the activity and other patients in the room. It was obvious we were the only "first timers." Most patients were asleep, fully reclined in their chairs. I knew my treatments would take hours to complete, but I did not like the idea of sleeping in an open room full of strangers. It somehow signaled to me a defeated state of mind. I told Manny I would never come to my appointments and just zone out. He agreed, as we shared sentiments on how precious every day is. I purposed in that moment to come to these appointments expecting to feel good and engage others. My Bible would be a priority, along with some research materials. I would take every opportunity to share my faith with anyone that would listen.

After the initial medications, it was time for my first chemotherapy infusion. Manny and I thought we were ready until we watched the nurse suit up. She transformed herself with a long-sleeve protective gown, complete with gloves, into a tightly wrapped cocoon. There was no need to ask why. It was obvious she could not afford to have any of the medication spill out onto her skin. Those drugs were powerful and, indeed, spilling the drug was not an option. Manny sent a text message to everyone at home, signaling my infusion had begun. We knew they would pray for us during this time. The next few hours seemed to pass slowly, as we patiently waited for each drug to complete the infusion process. Finally, my nurse indicated everything was complete, and it would take only minutes longer to disconnect the IV. She carefully reviewed my follow-up instructions and handed us a calendar showing all of my appointments for the next month. The entire infusion took over six hours, leaving both of us very anxious to return home.

Confessing I was tired from the whole ordeal, everyone acknowledged my need to rest. The following day brought words of reassurance and encouragement to try and eat something. However, even the thought of eating was difficult for me. I had already begun to feel the nauseating effects of the drugs. From this point, it took days before I could override those feelings, forcing myself to eat in order to gain some much-needed strength. Late at night seemed to be the worst, as I struggled to keep food down. Fortunately, after the first week this subsided, replaced only by incapacitating fatigue, brought on as the drugs worked against my blood cell count. During that time I had to be careful, as I was susceptible to infections. While I was made aware of the many possible side effects, it was something else to experience them. For instance, the fatigue could range from mild to debilitating. There were days when I did not have the strength to move from my bed to a chair without assistance or even hope to climb the stairs in my second-story house.

During that time, I found myself at the mercy of everyone, needing my family's help for just about everything. It was not easy for me to be in this position, but I learned to be gracious, accepting the help needed. Manny organized our home, shifting our kids into completely different roles. Brittany took over home schooling Jonathon and Timothy, while together they learned to take on most of the household chores. Sandy took over meal planning, assisted by Brittany, to include the goal of creating new and delicious ways to tempt me into eating strength-building foods. Beyond this, friends reached out and offered their support almost daily. My good friend Sheyla called on many occasions, offering to include the twins in her home schooling field trips, as well as other opportunities for them to spend time with her sons. On my better days, people stopped by to share a moment, giving me a hug and taking the time to pray. We experienced several powerful prayer meetings where God spoke expressly of healing. Nothing could replace the assurance God's presence brought in the midst of the believers.

By now, the winter months were fast approaching, leading us straight into the holiday season. Manny and I agreed it was somehow fitting, as I felt we were in the winter of my life. With Thanksgiving just around the corner, I began to see, regrettably, the need for Sandy to return home to her life in Florida. She had done an amazing job, helping me focus on my goal of alternative medicine and caring for my home as if it was her own. I had made the hard decision, encouraging her to return home in time to celebrate Thanksgiving with her husband, Bill. He, too, had contributed by patiently supporting Sandy's decision to stay in California for an undetermined length of time. Although it would be hard to see her go, it was time for us to manage things on our own. After all, she was just a phone call away. Saying goodbye at the airport meant holding onto her for as long as possible, letting tears fall, and realizing there were no words left to say. Manny and I hugged each other as we watched her disappear up the escalator.

My second round of chemotherapy fell during the week of Thanksgiving. As it turned out, most of the side effects were to be delayed until the next week, allowing me to at least enjoy this holiday. Temperatures outside began to shift, bringing a colder than usual forecast and providing an opportunity to light our fireplace. I really enjoyed cozying up to a warm fire after a long day at the medical center. By now I was into a weekly routine of infusion appointments, including lab and prep work. As promised, I went to each appointment dressed as nice as possible and bringing with me plenty of reading material. The nurses took notice and, with an open door, I shared my faith that God would heal me. I soon realized that exercising a positive attitude helped me avoid dreading those inevitable appointments. With only a few exceptions, I felt good and was able to engage others, hoping to invite someone to church or at least share words of encouragement. I was blessed every day to know the peace of God, and it was heart wrenching to have a front row seat to the suffering that cancer brings to patients and their loved ones.

In early December I stood in front of my bathroom mirror, brushing my hair and bending to pick up handfuls from off the floor. Slowly, I was loosing the battle to keep my beautiful, long hair. For now, there was only so much I could do to restyle the remaining hair in my attempt to cover the loss. While my sister was still staying with us, we had spent a little time shopping for a wig in preparation for this day. In fact, all three of us, Manny included, drove all over town stopping at almost every wig shop. Needless to say, we had some interesting experiences and a few laughs along the way. Eventually, I was able to find the perfect look that was similar to my original color and long length of hair. With that said, there was no easy way to confront the image in the mirror when all of my hair was gone. I experienced a deep sense of shame and feelings of guilt over the loss. The scariest thing was not being able to recognize myself. Besides the hair loss, I had dropped over twenty pounds, and a large horizontal scar stretched from under my right arm across the center of my chest. The reality was that I no longer looked like myself. As a woman, I had to fight the downside of my new image. Try as I did, everyday the mirror screamed back at me a message of doom. One day, late in December, I stepped from the shower into view of the mirror. Once again I stood there in disbelief, wanting to turn aside. Instead, I asked God to help me see past my reflection. While I finished dressing, He spoke a simple message that flooded my mind with these words, "Worship Me." The message was strong and compelling. Without hesitation I closed my eyes, freely worshipping God and giving back the love He had so often poured out on me. When I opened my eyes, I felt peace and a promise for future restoration.

It got to the point where I could track my progress by the next upcoming holiday. Christmas brought my third round of chemotherapy, marking the midway journey of my treatment. In some ways, I handled the treatments better each time, but the fatigue caused by a low-blood cell count was really taking a toll on my body. I began to notice a trend, waking up in the early morning hours with severe headaches. I started to medicate my headache praying they would simply fade away as easily as they appeared. When this did not happen, I called my oncologist to get her advice. Immediately she brought me in for an examination. After asking several questions she pushed back in her chair and recommended another MRI, stating my first scan only covered the torso area. In a very matter of fact voice, she estimated the cancer had most likely traveled to the region of the brain, causing the headaches. Upon hearing this, I made it clear there would be no additional MRI. Furthermore, I confidently told her the cancer had not traveled to my brain. At that moment, I spoke clearly from a place of faith, acting completely on God's promises. Accepting my response, she asked me to keep her informed on my condition. The next day I was scheduled for my weekly labs. These labs were available to my doctor within minutes of completing them. After arriving home I received a phone call, alerting me to an extremely low-blood cell count. I would have to undergo a blood transfusion to correct the issue. The good news was, as it turned out, that this was also the cause of my headaches.

It was January now, and my family was certainly glad to say goodbye to the old year. I had made it past the halfway mark in my treatment cycle with my latest CT scan, showing some improvements. It was time for my regular follow-up appointment with my oncologist. Since that next meeting was routine, I told Manny not to worry; I could handle this one on my own. So, once again, I drove to the medical center, where I sat in the oncologist office reviewing the status of my recent labs and my current infusion schedule. The only complication was a continuation of my low-blood cell count. This problem delayed my treatments and forced me to undergo additional blood transfusions. The source of the issue was simple. The chemotherapy drugs were just too hard on my body, confirming the need for an alternative plan. As my oncologist finished her review, it occurred to me that I had never asked her about my prognosis. Putting on a brave face, I posed the question to her. With a somewhat positive inflection in her voice, she revealed statistics would support a survival rate of less than one year. If those statistics were right, I would not see my next birthday. I followed this question by asking her how many women with a similar diagnosis had made it into remission. After pausing, she calculated her response by including everyone she had treated since 2006, choosing this year because of the available cancer drug, Herceptin. Apparently that drug had improved survival rates for women with breast cancer. Finally, she responded by telling me she had seen only three, possibly, four women into remission.

I fought the temptation to fall apart on my drive home. As much as those words frightened me, I could not give in to my emotions. I began to question why I had feelings of doubt. Clearly God had spoken to me, overshadowing any impact my doctor's words could have. Finally, I realized it was not about my doctor's words. It was God's words that mattered. The decision was mine to whom I would choose to listen to from this day forward. I reminded myself not to focus on her words, realizing the power they had to become my reality if allowed to be rehearsed over and over again. Manny had often expressed, in teaching Bible studies, that God was big on the power of the spoken word. I knew God had spoken, and I must act on His words alone.

Some time later, I shared with my Pastor's wife, Kim Haney, how I had come to terms with my survival statistic. She listened, as I shared how thoughts of despair and fear still returned to me. Although I would pray and redirect my thoughts, trying to focus on anything else, I struggled to put that behind me. After hearing me out, she shared what always worked for her when facing a spiritual battle. Out of her purse she pulled several note cards on which specific Scriptures were handwritten. She explained that she kept those verses handy, reading them whenever she needed strength. She reminded me that the Bible was a sword to be used offensively in my spiritual battle. I took this suggestion to heart and created my own cards. I took the time to laminate the cards and assemble them on a key ring. With these cards at hand, I would now be able to quote the Word against any thought contrary to God's promises. I began to use this strategy immediately, giving myself permission to reject negative thoughts and input from outside of God's Word. No longer would I be a victim held captive by thoughts of hopelessness. My future belonged in the hands of God, and I had learned to trust His Word coming to pass in my life.

God was involved in every detail of my life. He sustained me through my illness, orchestrating the answers I needed. My focus slowly shifted away from endless days of medical appointments to embrace an alternative way to regain my health. I had been walking for miles through the darkness of night, waiting for the rising sun to signal a new day. That day came when I committed to trust God completely for my healing. Convinced He had spoken to me through His Word and in prayer, I took every opportunity to thank God for my healing, well before it came. In God's own time He confirmed my healing. On April 10, 2011, our family went to church like we did every Sunday. I was so grateful to feel well enough on that day to attend. Worship was incredible, feeling God's presence move throughout the congregation,

I stepped out into the aisle continuing to lift up my voice in praise. I felt a strong pull toward the altar where others were gathering. As I moved forward a lady joined me, and we continued worshipping together. I was about halfway down the aisle when I experienced a feeling of cleansing throughout my body, accompanied by the sensation of being lighter than air. I had never felt this before, but I immediately knew God had brought healing to my body. In that moment, worshiping God was all that mattered.

The time had finally come for me to sever all ties to traditional medicine. My goal had always been to have an alternative plan in place by the time my chemotherapy ended. I promised never to return to those damaging treatments, believing there was a safer way to guard my health. Before moving forward, Manny and I had a very serious conversation that ensured we both understood the implications of my decision. Agreeing together, we chose to walk by faith, even unto death. There would be no turning back and no regrets. As soon as possible, Manny and I made an appointment with my oncologist. During this meeting, I shared my experience and choice to walk by faith, believing God would continue to keep me in His care. True to form, she showed very little emotion, as she acknowledged her concerns for my situation. She rehearsed several details about the aggressive nature of my particular cancer. Doing her best to remind me of the poor survival statistics, she advised me, at the very least, to undergo a CT scan. I was against any unnecessary exposure to radiation for I saw no need for imaging results. Manny, on the other hand, saw a great opportunity to prove I was indeed healed of cancer. With his encouragement, I agreed to the CT scan. Each day passed almost unnoticed as we waited for my results. My oncologist called late on a Friday afternoon and, in her same calm voice, relayed to us there was no evidence of cancer in the scan. Elated, we celebrated what God had done and shared the good news with everyone!

From that time forward I entered into a partnership with God, agreeing to protect my healing by following a healthy diet and lifestyle. I believed

God had placed healing power in the very foods He created. In their natural state, many foods possess the ability to cleanse, energize and heal the human body. I was determined to receive the blessing of good health by obeying what God had set in order for His creation.

Beloved, I wish above all things that thou mayest prosper and be in health, even as thy soul prospereth (III John 1:2).

PART TWO

My Challenge

Orthodox Versus Alternative Medicine

It is important to understand the vital role that nutrition plays in a person's overall health. Everyone has some idea of nutritional needs, but for many reasons people neglect their health through poor nutrition. Most people have heard the common phrase, "You are what you eat." However, do we really grasp the truth behind this statement? Statistics say otherwise. Figures on disease and chronic health issues in the United States are on the rise, even in the face of well-publicized, nutritional guidelines, leading to the conclusion that people do not understand the powerful connection between nutrition and their health.

It is apparent with the rise in medical research and advancements we have come to rely on a "prescription-based" answer for healthcare. As a whole, people are now programmed to expect medication to solve any health problem. The pharmaceutical industry operates on the success of this belief system. In 2004, a study by two York University researchers, Marc-Andre Gagnon and Joel Lexchin, estimated the U.S. pharmaceutical industry spends almost twice as much on promotion as it does on research. "The researchers' estimate is based on the systematic collection of data directly from the industry and doctors during 2004, which shows the U.S. pharmaceutical industry spent 24.4% of the sales dollar on promotion, versus 13.4% for research and development, as a percentage of US domestic sales of US$235.4 billion."[1] This information is staggering and should help us understand who profits in the promotion of drugs as the frontline solution in healthcare. The study's findings support the idea that this industry is marketing-driven, instead of a research-driven, life-saving, industry. In addition, this same idea can be applied to individual, disease-focused research organizations that claim to be in search of a "cure." Year after year, millions of dollars are donated to these organizations under the assumption that someday funding for research will result in a cure; however, a quick search on these websites for the word "cure" produces zero results. Instead, the content of these websites focuses entirely on the ongoing solicitation for the funding of a host of specialized research projects. Professionals, political and entertainment personalities, industry leaders, and every form of media available support these organizations. They operate by appealing to the most vulnerable people – the patient and their families, who desperately want to believe a cure is possible.

Based on the above information, a person must ask why modern medicine has not been able to produce a cure for cancer and other chronic diseases in the twenty-first century. There certainly is enough money pouring into every imaginable area of research. Still, more and more people are diagnosed each year, and we are no closer to a cure then we were more than fifty years ago. Yes, cancer has been around for many years. In the same amount of time, we have seen the development of vaccines to prevent chicken pox, diphtheria, malaria, measles, pertussis (whooping cough), pneumococcal disease, polio, tetanus, typhoid fever, and smallpox.[2] Vaccines have eradicated many diseases from most parts of the world. It is difficult to accept that well-funded medical and pharmaceutical industries together with many brilliant scientists worldwide, have not developed a cure for cancer. Perhaps, they are searching for the wrong answers. Is it possible that instead of searching for a cure, they should be searching for a cause?

Should research focus on the cure or the cause of cancer? This is not a new idea. In fact, it is a recurring theme throughout all the research I have found concerning traditional medicine versus natural or alternative medicine. These two schools of thought are polar opposites. Traditional or orthodox medicine operates from the standpoint that a "cure" can only arise out of a drug created in a laboratory. This leads us once again to the lucrative pharmaceutical industry that is funded by the expensive "patented" drugs they create. The healthcare industry rejects the idea that natural medicine produces results. However, imagine what would happen if, through natural medicine, a person could be cured of cancer or other diseases. The pharmaceutical industry would lose its multi-billion dollar business. In addition, millions of dollars would be lost to the healthcare industry because support facilities, medical personnel and technology would no longer be needed. This observation points to two distinct points of view. Traditional medicine seeks after a cure through funding drug research. Natural medicine seeks after the cause of the disease. Natural medicine understands that if you identify the cause, you have a path to the cure.

What Causes Cancer?

This brings up the question of what causes cancer. If you ask an oncologist, as I did, you will be told that no one really knows. On the other hand, alternative medicine has a wealth of well-defined information on this subject. In the simplest of terms, an imbalance between the strength of the immune system and the number of cancer cells in a person's body causes cancer. Every person gets new cancer cells all the time, but for most people their immune systems safely kill these new cancer cells. God has designed our bodies to do just this. However, if the immune system is weak or the cancer cells grow out of control, then the person is diagnosed with cancer.[3] Logically, the way to treat cancer is by restoring the immune system and safely targeting and killing cancer cells.

The medical industry agrees that cancer cells must be targeted and killed, but they do not agree on restoring the immune system or safely killing the cancer cells. Typically, a cancer patient will be given the option of one or more of these major treatments: surgery, radiation, and chemotherapy. These treatments either remove or are designed to kill fast-growing cells. The problem is that certain normal, healthy cells also grow quickly and cancer treatments affect these cells, too. The cells most likely to be affected are blood-forming cells in the bone marrow, as well as cells in the digestive track, reproductive system, and hair follicles.[4] When this happens it is an indicator that the treatment is toxic to the body. Many of the known side effects to chemotherapy attest to this fact. For example, the patient undergoes complete loss of his/her hair. While this is emotionally devastating, it is even more devastating to comprehend what is taking place inside the body. Other serious side effects may include loss of appetite, nausea and vomiting, fatigue, anemia, burning and numbing pain in the hands and feet, skin and nail problems, diarrhea, sterilization, cognitive impairment, and depression, just to mention a few. At the very minimum, the immune system, stomach lining, and colon are all compromised.[5] These three systems are critical to fight cancer. In addition, not all cancer cells are fast growing, so certain cancer cells may not be killed with these treatments.

Not all cancer patients are the same. Depending on the stage of cancer, treatments may appear to be working, but the patients immune systems are nevertheless greatly damaged. The ability to digest and extract nutrients from food is nearly impossible due to a damaged stomach lining and colon. Unless a long-term plan is established that rebuilds the immune system and restores other vital functions, the cancer patients will face a recurrence of their cancer.[6] To further emphasize, before patients enter treatment, their oncologist will tell them that it is impossible to kill every cancer cell in the body. This sets the patients up for an ongoing cycle of future treatment. Why? Initially, the cancer cells may be killed by the treatment, but the natural defenses for healing the body are undermined and in this condition the body will at some point experience a return of the cancer. It is very simple, whichever is stronger, the cancer or the body's defenses, will win.

WHY CHOOSE ALTERNATIVE TREATMENTS?

My circumstances were different than most newly-diagnosed cancer patients. Initially, I was told that my cancer was detected early, but soon after my biopsy, the cancer grew at an alarming rate due to the HER2-positive factor. This meant that I had no time to do research, much less think about treatment options. Unfortunately, I chose orthodox treatment, believing at the time this was my only choice. I was well into accepting orthodox treatment when I heard about alternative medicine. Immediately, I began to gather information on this topic. The idea of treating my cancer naturally and safely was an answer to prayer.

Primarily, I used the Internet, magazines, local bookstores and the library to obtain information. I also made phone calls to hospitals and clinics, both in and outside the United States. I set up a file folder to help me organize the information and to make it readily accessible. Please understand, this did not happen overnight. During that time, I had already had surgery and was in chemotherapy treatment. Needless to say, there were plenty of days, and even weeks, when I was too sick to do anything. In spite of this, I knew that God had placed me on this path. I was driven by His confirmation in my spirit that this would lead to vital answers. It was like piecing together a picture puzzle, knowing the end result would be something beautiful. From this experience, I learned that the most important thing a cancer patient could do is to conduct research before agreeing to any treatment.

I cannot stress enough the importance of reading and comparing information. A key thing to look for and document is when you discover the same information showing up in multiple sources. This indicates that the information is widely accepted and supported by reliable research. This type of information will become foundational in your treatment decisions. In addition, the more you search, the more likely it is for you to discover critical information for your specific type of cancer. For example, while searching for causes of cancer, I happened upon a website devoted to breast cancer. This site provided well-documented data supporting the idea that women with breast cancer were found to have low levels of iodine.[7] Sure enough, my own blood work revealed that I was low in iodine. I then researched iodine and breast cancer. I quickly found a host of information confirming the need for women to maintain adequate levels of iodine as a defense against breast cancer. I concluded that taking an iodine supplement would be an important part of my treatment plan.

I continued to apply this same strategy as I searched to understand alternative versus orthodox treatment. Slowly, I began to see a much bigger picture in which I was dealing. The information coming from both sides was indeed at opposite ends of the medical spectrum. I found a few, rare cases where certain hospitals had begun to integrate alternative treatments into their otherwise orthodox plans. I found no support from inside or outside of my own healthcare system. In fact, I discovered that living in the state of California would prove to be a detriment to any choice outside of orthodox medicine. For example, I learned that infusing a cancer patient with high doses of vitamin C and oxygen would kill cancer cells. Excited about this news, I contacted several private practices in my area that offered these treatments. Each time I attempted to schedule an appointment, I was promptly rejected upon finding out that I was a cancer patient. I was stunned the first few times this happened, but finally I made up my mind that I would push for an answer. So, I called yet another office, and again I was denied an appointment. Refusing to get off the phone, I begged a nurse to tell me why I could not have those treatments. After hesitating, she told me that the state of California passed legislation making it illegal for a medical doctor to talk to a cancer patient about any treatment other than chemotherapy.

This was not the only obstacle I faced. I had also begun to search for an oncologist that practiced alternative medicine. In fact, I was looking for any kind of physician that practiced alternative medicine. However, my search turned up zero options in California. Finally, the picture came into clearer focus. Our country's healthcare system had cornered the market in cancer treatment by using the legal system to force every other medical professional out of business or out of the country.

After coming to terms with this and realizing that I was not in a position to leave the country to find treatment, I turned all of my efforts into continuing my own research with the idea of piecing together a workable treatment plan. I was convinced that God would heal me and that He would lead me to seek natural treatment that would prove to be a plan for life. With this understanding, I knew that I was going to move forward in faith, choosing to leave orthodox treatment behind.

PART THREE

My Plan

The intricate functioning of our own bodies is something of a marvel. We are wonderfully complex and a testament of God's handy work. He has carefully designed all the systems of our bodies to work together to achieve their intended objective of our survival. God is also the creator of what our bodies need to remain healthy and function at their optimum.

This leads me to the important topic of what fuels our body – food. In their natural state, many foods are powerful agents in the arena of good health. God has actually designed certain foods to fight and protect our bodies against disease. For a cancer patient, this is good news. The ability to carefully provide our bodies with proper nutrition makes all the difference. Fortunately, we are empowered with the gift of choice.

To make good choices you need to understand what is important to obtain good nutrition. In today's terms, you must eat only what is natural, and this means organic. By definition, organic foods are produced without synthetic pesticides and chemical fertilizers. In addition, you must exclude all foods that are contrary to your goal of healing. The Standard American Diet (SAD) primarily consists of too many processed meats, dairy products, carbohydrates, refined sugars and starches, oils, caffeine, alcohol, etc. These foods are off limits to the cancer patient. You will have to be committed to eating only what is designed to equip your body in the process of healing.

The list of foods you can eat have been carefully selected for their cancer-fighting properties. As I mentioned above, you must be diligent in sticking to these approved foods, while avoiding all other foods. Adding anything to this list can prove to be a setback in your healing. For instance, carrot juice is a powerful cancer-fighting vegetable.[8] However, it contains a lot of natural sugar. Sugar is the number one food source for cancer cells. In the case of the carrot juice, the cancer cell readily absorbs the juice due to the sugar content, but then the carotenoids in the carrot juice kill the cancer cell. This is only possible when all other sugar in the patient's diet is eliminated. Otherwise, additional sugar in the patient's diet will continue to feed cancer cells present in the body.[9]

The best thing you can do is to practice reading ingredients on packaging labels. This will help you to become aware of the harmful and unnecessary ingredients in almost every food item. A good rule of thumb: If you cannot pronounce or recognize the ingredient, you should not be eating it. Take time to compare similar foods that are non-organic to those that are organic. You will be amazed to see all of the artificial preservatives, coloring, flavorings, etc. in the non-organic items.

Now that I have explained the importance of organic foods, it is time to look at the treatment plan that I chose. My research revealed that alternative treatment plans always include a main protocol, plus several additional secondary protocols or treatments. The idea behind this is to provide as much support as possible to the cancer-fighting objective. Keep in mind that there are many different protocols to choose from, as they relate to a particular type of cancer. While I am confident in the one I am presenting here, it was chosen as a primary treatment for Stage IV breast cancer. Although this same plan works for pancreatic, gallbladder, liver and lung cancers, it is advisable that you do your own research to be sure of your decision. For this reason, I have provided a resource section at the end of this book. The information there will be valuable to your research. Finally, carefully read all of the information in the treatment plan. I have purposely presented each step in two parts. First, the "goal" provides instruction on the treatment. Second, the "supporting details" give specific information on the importance of the treatment. It is important to remember that all of the following steps are crucial, as they add up to a comprehensive protocol.

Pure Drinking Water

◆ Goal

Every day you will need to set a goal to drink half your body weight in ounces.[10] For example, a person who weights 120 lbs. would drink 60 ounces of water. You may also include your vegetable juicing in this daily liquid count.

To insure that your drinking water is pure, you will need to invest in a water purification system. I chose to use a reverse osmosis system. This system guarantees the highest contaminant removal rates, giving me the purest water possible. Manny installed this system under the kitchen sink, providing our whole family with a continuous source of pure water in which to drink and to cook. There are many online sources available to purchase a reverse osmosis system. I have included the company that I purchased my system from in the resource section of this book. If you choose a reverse osmosis system, be sure to purchase the filter that adds minerals back into the water. Essential minerals are remove during the filtration process. Please note there are other types of systems available. Once again, you will need to do your own research in order to be sure of the best choice for you.

◆ Supporting Details

Why pure drinking water? Water is a life-giving source. It is essential for every function of the human body. It is, therefore, important that you drink enough water and that the water you drink is pure. Unfortunately, the time has come that our drinking water, including city systems, lakes, rivers, and even glaciers, contain levels of contamination. Contaminants range from natural minerals to industrial chemicals and by-products.[11] You may drink bottled water, which should have a better quality than city or tap water. However, the fact is that bottled water sold in the United States is not always filtered and not necessarily cleaner or safer than most tap water. This is according to a four-year scientific study recently made public by the Natural Resources Defense Council (NRDC).[12] You also have to consider the adverse effects of drinking from plastic bottles that leach chemicals into the water. It is advisable that you drink only from glass or stainless steel containers. Severe illnesses including, liver damage and cancer are proven to occur from low-level exposure to contaminants.

The importance of pure water cannot be overstated. Water supports many of the basic mechanics of the human body. Water is needed for everything from detoxifying to regulating the temperature of our body. The human body weight is comprised of more than two-thirds water. Without water, we would die in a few days. Our brain is made up of 95% water; lungs are 90% water and blood is 82%. A 2% drop in our body's water level can result in signs of dehydration: short-term memory loss, trouble with basic calculations, and trouble focusing on a computer screen. One of the most common causes of fatigue is mild dehydration. Almost three-fourths of Americans suffer from mild, chronic dehydration.[13]

A Raw Food Diet and Juicing

◆ Goal

You will set a goal to primarily eat and/or juice fresh, raw vegetables and fruits each day. You will choose from a very select group of vegetables and fruits. These vegetables and fruits are categorized as having nutrients that kill cancer cells. In addition, they help to build a strong immune system.

Your raw food diet is an exclusive diet and must be adhered to strictly. This means what you eat is just as important as what you do not eat. To be successful, you must not eat certain foods, such as meat, poultry, fish, dairy products, refined sugars, starches, carbohydrates, and vegetables oils. To be more specific, there should be no cooked meats, fat, butter, margarine, eggs, milk, cheese, salad dressings, potatoes, breads, bakery goods, etc. All of these food categories have contributing factors for cancer. For instance, drinking cow's milk into adulthood has been linked to Type 1 diabetes, breast cancer, overweight, gastrointestinal problems, and prostate cancer.[14] The reason for restricting your diet is two-fold. Cooked foods are more difficult to digest, tasking the immune system, while it is needed to fight cancer. Also, foods high in starches and sugar dilute the amount of cancer-killing nutrients that enter the cancer cell, making the treatment less effective. Remember, sugar fuels the cancer cell.[15]

Although the list of restrictions is limiting, there are plenty of foods you can enjoy that are healthy for your diet. The key is to learn what foods you can substitute to help round out your meal plan. It is necessary for most people to rethink and retrain their taste buds to enjoy a whole new way of eating. If you have spent a lifetime eating mostly processed, prepared foods, then your taste buds crave salt, sugar, and a chemical-based diet. For the most part, you have been eating "dead" foods, lacking nutritional value. Your goal now is to eat "live" foods that are rich in nutrients.

Below are just a few ideas of healthy substitutes in a raw food diet.

1. Organic rice or almond milk instead of cow milk.
2. Sprouted grain bread instead of "enriched" wheat flour bread. Sprouted grains have increased vitamin and nutrient content because the seed is first sprouted, making it alive in its growth process.[16] Sprouted grains are available in a variety of products, including cereals, pasta, tortillas, etc.
3. Organic olive oil instead of vegetable oils, fats, salad dressings, butter or margarine. This is the only other oil you can use outside of organic flaxseed oil. It is great for sauteing vegetables on a low-heat setting.

4. Organic brown rice and pastas, instead of white. Brown rice is the whole grain with just the first outer layer (husk or hull) removed through milling. It retains its fiber and germ, which contain vital nutrients.[17]

VEGETABLES

There is overwhelming research that supports the cancer-fighting ability in the group of vegetables I included in my diet. The vegetables you should focus on are carrots, cabbage, green asparagus, broccoli, kale, swiss shard, red beets (i.e. beetroot), beet tops, cauliflower and related cruciferous vegetables. I would like to make specific mention about carrots. I have read many documented cases where carrots were used exclusively to fight cancer. The power of carrots lies in the group of pigments called carotenoids (beta-carotene is among this group), which give them their orange color. Most important characteristic is their antioxidant capability. Carotenoids can directly scavenge free radicals and fight cancer through vitamin A by promoting normal cell differentiation.[18]

By far the best way to eat vegetables is to juice. There are two advantages to juicing. First, juicing makes the nutrients in a fruit or vegetable more digestible by the body and removes fibers that obstruct this process. Second, you can consume a larger amount of foods in a shorter amount of time. It is important that you drink your juice as soon as you complete the juicing process. Enzymes and other nutrients have a short life and must be consumed immediately.[19]

My daily amount of juicing included:

1. Carrot juice – 1 to 2 quarts
2. Vegetables – 1 to 2 quarts of broccoli, cabbage, cauliflower, swiss chard, kale and 2 red beets with their leafy stem and tops
3. Green apple – Add one to any of your juices

When shopping for vegetables, choose the freshest and darkest colors available. Every part of the vegetable is nutritious. This means you will want to use everything from the leaves to the root, including the stems. In many cases, there is more nutritional value in the leaves and stems than any other part of the plant.

Recommended

1. Try adding a small amount of organic apple cider vinegar to your vegetable juice for flavor and additional health benefits. Be sure and use only raw unfiltered apple cider vinegar. In the fermentation process, it produces enzymes, bacteria and life-giving nutrients. You can actually see it settled in the bottom of the bottle. These beneficial ingredients help you to feel more energized. It is reported to help regulate blood pressure, reduce bad cholesterol, create strong bones, maintain proper pH levels, and prevent brittle teeth, hair loss and runny noses, just to mention a few.[20] I purchase my organic apple cider vinegar from a health food store.
2. You can super charge your juice by adding a number of healthy products. The two that I recommend are organic spirulina and liquid chlorophyll. Spirulina boosts your immune system and is a complete vegetarian protein, which is essential for this treatment plan. It is around 65% protein, making it greater gram for gram than red meat and soy.[21] Chlorophyll directly affects hemoglobin. It helps to rebuild and replenish red blood cells, providing the energy your body needs.[22] I include additional information on these products in the supplement section.

FRUITS

There is also a group of fruits that can help fight cancer. Just like the vegetables, this group is limited, due to the high fructose content of many fruits. It is important that you eliminate sugar from every area of your diet.

The good news is that there is no limit to how many fruit juices you can have each day.

You should focus on dark colored fruits. Clinical studies have confirmed these fruits have an inhibiting effect on specific cancers.[23] Purple grapes (with skins and seeds), red raspberries, black raspberries, strawberries, blueberries, and other non-citrus fruits with their seeds, especially peaches and apricots (the seed is inside a hard shell) are among my favorites.[24] Also, raw pineapple and tomatoes have cancer-fighting nutrients. In addition, you are allowed mangosteen, noni and wolfberry or goji. These are considered super-fruit juices and can be enjoyed in unlimited quantities.

Purchasing a Juicer

In this section, I will discuss guidelines for selecting a juicer. Not all juicers are alike, so you must consider the purpose behind juicing in your decision. The main thing you want to accomplish is to preserve the important enzymes and other nutrients in your juice. In order to do this, you need to purchase a single-gear masticating, a twin-gear juicer or a grind and press machine. You need to avoid a centrifugal juicer for the reasons covered below. After comparing juicers, I chose to buy an Omega 8003 single-gear masticating juicer. This juicer met all of my nutritional requirements, as well as being a good match for my budget. It is also easy to clean. This is an important feature, as you will be juicing many times a day. Below is a brief description of the different types of juicers. As with all products mentioned in this book, the best thing to do is to research and price compare online.

1. Masticating Juicers – single gear
   This juicer uses a single gear or auger to chew fruit and vegetable fibers. They turn at slow speeds, preserving vital nutrients. This breaks up plant cells, yielding more fiber, enzymes, vitamins and trace minerals. They

can juice virtually any fruit or vegetable, as well as extract juice from wheatgrass, swiss shard, kale, and other leafy greens. This juicer is easy to clean.[25]

2. Twin-gear Juicers

   Twin-gear juicers turn at even slower speeds than masticating juicers. They are an efficient juicer able to extract high yields of juice from fruits, vegetables, wheatgrass, and other greens. This juicer operates by pressing food between two interlocking roller gears. This juicing process yields a larger volume of juice. The high pressure squeezing force of the twin-gears breaks open tough cell walls and releases more enzymes, vitamins and trace minerals.[26]

2. Grind and Press Juicers

   This is a two-step machine, with a grinder and a hydraulic press. The food is first ground into a fine pulp. Second, the press extracts the juice under high pressure. This two-step process yields the maximum amount of juice leaving the extracted pulp dry. This juicer is highly efficient in releasing enzymes and minerals.[27] However, it is also very expensive.

4. Centrifugal Juicers

   These juicers first grate the fruit or vegetable into a pulp, and then use centrifugal force to push the pulp against a strainer screen by spinning it at a very high RPM. The problem with this juicer is that the high speed generates heat and aerates the juice. The heat kills the enzymes and other nutrients. For this reason, this type of juicer is not recommended.[28]

◆ Supporting Details

Why is it necessary to choose a raw food diet? Raw foods are considered live foods because they contain important enzymes, electrons and biophotons.

First, enzymes are needed to digest food and to get nutrients out of food. Foods that are heated at a temperature above 105 degrees will destroy 100% of all enzymes. Next, raw foods are electron rich. Electrons in raw foods are provided as stored energy from the sun. The more electrons you have in the body, the more energy for healing and proper functioning of all systems. All of this points to the fact that we are "body electric." In other words, we are electromagnetic. Our bodies contain somewhere between 60 and 100 trillion cells. These cells fire electrically. The center of each cell is positively charged and the cell membrane is negatively charged. Each cell is a little electromagnetic field, which fires at about -70 to -90 millivolts dc in our body. Now imagine the energy available when all 60 to 100 trillion cells are firing. The available energy we have directly correlates to our ability to obtain the sun's energy from the foods we eat. When we fail to eat raw foods, we knock down the electrical charge in our bodies. If the electrical charge drops to -50 mV or -40 mV, you will feel tired and lethargic. However, if this electrical charge drops to around -30 mV, you most certainly will have cancer. Finally, biophotons are the smallest physical units of sunlight which our cells must have. When you are eating an apple or carrot, you are eating pure sunlight. These biophotons travel in wavelengths from cell to cell throughout the body. They have an important part in creating order and transmitting information between the cells. It also appears that this light energy is stored in your DNA. It is believed that the higher the level of light energy a cell emits, the greater the transfer of energy to the person. The more light a food is able to store, the more energy and vitality transferred to the person. The cells absorb light into the nucleolus, and then your cells emit this light back out.[29]

One final thought, when cells are healthy, they use a process called aerobic respiration. This is a process of cellular respiration that uses oxygen in order to break down molecules, releasing electrons and creating energy. When this happens, aerobic respiration creates a substance known as adenosine triphosphate (ATP). This is responsible for storing and carrying most of the energy to other body cells, thus making it possible for life to continue.[30] The cells and tissues are oxygen rich. However, when people eat the typical Standard American Diet (SAD) their cells become acidic, and this acid pushes the oxygen out of the cells. When the oxygen is pushed out of the cell, the cell becomes anaerobic, firing off sugar, glucose, fermentation and lactic acid. As a result, a person develops cancer. This does not happen overnight but through years of depriving the body of both hydration and proper nutrition.[31] Chemists express the degree of acidity or alkalinity on the pH scale that runs from about 0 to 14. Acidic solutions have pH values of less than 7, alkaline solutions more than 7. Pure water, being neutral, has a pH of exactly 7. Establishing the proper pH of your body is critical. Most people that are dealing with a chronic illness have a body pH of around 4.5 to 5.5.[32] This means that they are acidic. You can check your own pH by using pH test papers. These can be purchased online or at most health stores. Ideally, you want your body to be slightly alkaline. Your urine pH should be about 6.8 to 7. You can increase the pH of your body through drinking pure water and eating a raw food diet.

THE BUDWIG PROTOCOL

◆ GOAL

To add the Budwig mixture of flaxseed oil and cottage cheese to your daily diet. Purchase only organic flaxseed oil without lignan, as well as organic cottage cheese. These two ingredients must be properly combined, using a hand blender, and not simply stirred together. It is important to bind the oil with the protein so that it becomes water-soluble and can enter the bloodstream. When they are blended, by using the low speed on your blender, the mixture will have the consistency of a thick pudding.

The recipe below calls for a two-to-one ratio of cottage cheese to flaxseed oil. The recommended daily consumption is between six and eight tablespoons of flaxseed oil for a person with cancer. You must consume the mixture fresh each time you blend it.[33] Due to the amazing health benefits, I continue to use this recipe once a day to maintain my health.

Flaxseed Oil and Cottage Cheese Recipe (twice daily)
1. Six to eight tablespoons of organic cottage cheese
2. Three to four tablespoons of organic flaxseed oil without lignan

You can find a video on Youtube by typing in "Budwig Recipe."

Optional Toppings

Only use the following items as toppings. Do not add while blending the flaxseed oil and cottage cheese. You can use any type of organic fruit, or possibly different organic nuts, like almonds and pecans. Also, consider a topping of organic sunflower seeds or ground organic pumpkin seeds. You can stir in organic cocoa, organic shredded coconut, organic cinnamon, or (freshly) squeezed organic fruit juice to add flavor. I always include a topping of freshly-ground organic flaxseeds. These can be purchased at your local health food store. I simply grind them in a coffee grinder and add to the mixture. This protocol makes an excellent breakfast item.

◆ Supporting Details

Dr. Johanna Budwig was born in Germany in 1908. She was a top European Cancer Research Scientist, Biochemist, Blood Specialist, German Pharmacologist, and Physicist. She was a seven-time Nobel Prize nominee.[34]

Dr. Budwig was one of the world's leading authorities on fats and oils. She discovered that blood from a healthy person contained greater amounts of Omega 3 essential fatty acids than blood samples from someone who was ill. Her research proved the harmful effects that commercially-processed fats and oils plus, hydrogenated fats, have in destroying cell membranes and lowering the voltage of the cells in our bodies. The cooking oils found on the shelves of your local grocer are extracted from corn, sunflowers, plants, etc., by using extreme heat and chemicals. They are no longer alive but are dead oils that have a 20-year shelf life.[35] As a result, their unsaturated qualities have been destroyed and the field of electrons removed. As we have discussed, without the charge, our cells lose oxygen and start to suffocate. Remember, we are "body electric." Dr Budwig discovered that modern processing of fats and oils destroys the field of electrons that the cell membranes in our bodies must have to fire properly. This affects every function of our bodies. For instance, when cells divide, the cell and the new daughter cell must contain enough-electron rich fatty acids on the membrane surface to divide completely. The highly-processed fats and oils in today's foods render this process inactive, which results in the formation of tumors.[36] Keep in mind, these same processed fats and oils are also included in many foods, ranging from canned goods to bakery items.

In her research, Dr. Budwig discovered that flaxseed oil has essential electron-rich unsaturated fats. Furthermore, she discovered that when combined with the sulfur protein in cottage cheese, the oil became water soluble and easily absorbed into the cell membrane. This caused the reversal of the cell's inability to function and divide properly. Dr. Budwig used her theory of flaxseed oil and cottage cheese to successfully treat patients with cancer and other diseases. Dr. Budwig used her protocol to treat other chronic diseases, such as arthritis, heart infarction, irregular heart beat, psoriasis, eczema (other skin diseases), immune deficiency syndromes (multiple sclerosis and other auto immune diseases), diabetes, lungs (respiratory conditions), stomach ulcers, liver, prostate, strokes, brain tumors, brain (strengthens activity), arteriosclerosis and other chronic diseases. This treatment proved successful, where orthodox, traditional medicine failed.[37]

SUPPLEMENTS

◆ GOAL

To carefully determine your need for supplements. Supplements can inhibit cancer. They work to assist the body's defense mechanisms to block metastatic cancer and prevent recurrences.[38] By definition, supplements complete a nutritional need where there is a deficiency. I recommend that you contact your doctor and request lab work that will provide your current levels of essential vitamins and minerals. You can review this information to determine where you are deficient. In addition, I also strongly recommend that you read as much as possible about the body's need for vitamins and minerals in relation to fighting disease. From your research, you will create a specific list of supplements to buy. It is important that you purchase organic whole food vitamins. Adding quality supplements to your diet will greatly ensure the success of your campaign for good health.

There is another option to explore. After reviewing your lab results and independent research, consider using a product that provides a wide range of nutritional supplements. One such product is called "Cellect." This product is available for purchase online. Be sure to read all the information provided, concerning this product, at www.cancertutor.com under Complete Protocols: Cellect–Budwig.

◆ SUPPORTING DETAILS

Vitamins and minerals are necessary at the cellular level to maintain a healthy body. With all the concern over nutrition, it is no wonder that most people are not getting the proper amounts of essential vitamins and minerals. With this said, supplements do not replace good nutrition. Instead, they support, or partner, with your nutrition effort to ensure your body performs at its best.

Today, there is increasing evidence that supplements can help to prevent future health concerns. Many researchers find that some important vitamins and minerals are also protective against disease. Even if we are conscientious about our diet, it may be difficult to obtain the right amount of vitamins and minerals needed to defend our bodies against disease.[39] For this reason alone, I highly recommend taking supplements.

After reviewing my lab results and reading extensively, I chose to purchase individual supplements to complete my nutritional needs. Below is a list of these supplements and a brief explanation of each one's importance to the overall picture of my health. You can find additional information on each one by further conducting your own research.

1. Iodine

   In the United States, the average person's intake of iodine has decreased by 50% over the past 36 years. Changes in the American diet are contributing factors. There is evidence to support that maintaining optimum levels of iodine in the body will lower the risk of cancer and fibrocystic disease of the breast.[40]

2. Moducare

   This product enhances a weak immune system and regulates an overactive one. A strong immune system is critical in fighting illness and disease.[41]

3. Coenzyme-A

   This product is a "master enzyme" supporting the production of cellular energy, detoxification, fatty acid metabolism, the reduction of stress and the support of the immune system.[42]

4. ToCoQ10

   Coenzyme Q10 (CoQ10) is a fat-soluble, vitamin-like compound found in every cell of the body. It is used by the cell to produce energy. It is found, in its highest concentration in cells of organs that require large amounts of energy, like the heart. It provides cardiovascular support and antioxidant protection.[43]

5. Spirulina

   Spirulina is a blue-green algae. It is a complete vegetarian protein and source of healthy, essential fatty acids. It is rich in amino acids, carotenoids, chlorophyll, minerals, and vitamins, that in combination, support the immune system, provide antioxidant defense and promote healthy circulation.[44]

6. Selenium

   Selenium is a trace mineral. It is an essential component of glutathione, the body's most potent natural antioxidant. It is a cancer preventive exhibiting abilities to end free radicals as confirmed in 55 studies reviewed by Cornell University and University of California researchers.[45]

7. Vitamin B-100 Complex

   This is a combination of essential B vitamins, which supports healthy cell function and energy production. They are referred to as "stress vitamins," helping to release energy from foods, aid the metabolic process and produce red blood cells.[46]

8. Calcium with magnesium

   Calcium promotes healthy bones and magnesium contributes to calcium absorption.[47]

9. Zinc

   Zinc is a trace mineral essential for proper growth, development and reproduction, as well as numerous body processes. It is also required for the proper function of approximately 300 enzymes. Zinc is necessary for the formation of superoxide dismutase (SOD), which is an important free radical scavenger in the body. It is also an antioxidant, meaning it helps protect healthy cells from the potentially damaging effects of free radicals.[48]

10. Chromium
    Chromium is an essential trace mineral required for normal protein, fat and carbohydrate metabolism.[49]

11. Branch Chain Amino Acids
    BCAAs support muscle tissue by preventing breakdown and maintain lean muscle mass.[50]

12. Mega Digestive Enzymes with Pancreatin 10X
    Provides enzymes important for digestion and the absorption of nutrients. They are essential to the breakdown of carbohydrates, protein and fats.[51]

13. Vitamin E
    Because vitamin E is an antioxidant, it can reduce the damage that free radicals cause to the body. It supports eye health and a strong blood system.[52]

14. Turmeric
    Turmeric contains a mixture of powerful phytonutrients, known as curcuminoids. Promotes healthy liver function and powerful, free radical scavenging activity. It is a strong cancer-fighter shown to help prevent breast cancer.[53]

15. Vitamin D3

    Vitamin D supports the maintenance of healthy bones and teeth, cellular function and the proper function of the immune and nervous systems. It is also important in fighting the development of colon, breast, and prostate cancers.[54] Vitamin D3 is the same Vitamin D that the body makes when the skin is exposed to natural sunlight. It is available in very few foods.

16. Vitamin A

    This vitamin helps maintain cell membranes by inhibiting the start of infectious diseases. Vitamin A fights cancer by blocking the production of DNA in cancerous cells. It also retards tumor growth in established cancer.[55] Vitamin A plays an important role in proper bone formation, reproduction and vision.

17. Liquid Chlorophyll

    Chlorophyll is almost identical to the molecular structure of hemoglobin. Taking chlorophyll increases the number of red blood cells, and this increases oxygen utilization by the body. It also is highly alkaline, providing many health benefits that include anti-carcinogenic, antioxidant, and chelation of heavy metals, just to mention a few.[56]

Holistic Detoxification

◆ Goal

To perform all necessary steps to detox the colon, gallbladder, liver and tissues, allowing all systems in the body to focus on the healing process. It is important that you follow these recommendations precisely in the order they are given. Every step is designed to stimulate the release of waste and debris from your body.[57] You can find the materials needed at a local health store or online at a nutritional supplement store.

1. Colon Cleanse

   Materials: Wheat germ oil, Sonne's® # 7 (bentonite clay), Sonne's® # 9 (psyllium powder), Barley green tablets, Beet juice tablets, Vitamin C (l,000 mg), Herbal laxative, Pint jar or large cup, Your choice of juice

The colon cleanse should be done for seven days. You may do it fasting, with only water, in addition to the tablets and drink above. This is very difficult to do for seven days for most people. You may do a liquid or juice fast instead. If you do choose to juice, please don't use any juices with high fructose corn syrup. Use only 100% organic juice. Preferably, you should make your own juice. Include more vegetable juices than fruit juices to avoid excess sugar intake. You may choose to do liquids with one meal of vegetables and fruit a day. Drink at least one gallon of water a day. Everything you eat should be organic. You cannot have any dairy products or meat products. In all cases, use only reverse osmosis or distilled water.[58]

Drink

1. Pour one inch of juice into the jar.
2. Add at least 10 ounces of water
3. Add 1 tablespoon of Sonne's® #7 (bentonite clay)
4. Add 1 teaspoon of Sonne's® #9 (psyllium powder)
5. Put cover on and shake vigorously for 12-15 seconds.
6. Drink quickly, as it gels fast.

Supplements

Wheat germ oil . . . . . . .One capsule
Barley green . . . . .Six tablets
Vitamin C . . . . .one tablet

Beet juice . . . . .Two tablets
Laxative . . . . .One to two at night IF needed.

Schedule

1. 7:00 am . . . . .Drink
2. 8:30 am . . . . .Supplements
3. 10:00 am . . . . .Drink
4. 11:30 am . . . . .Supplements
5. 1:00 pm . . . . .Drink
6. 2:30 pm . . . . .Supplements
7. 4:00 pm . . . . .Drink
8. 5:30 pm . . . . .Supplements

If you weigh over 150 lbs.

9. 7:00 pm . . . . .Drink
10. 8:30 pm . . . . .Supplements

After the first one to two days, you should be having multiple bowel movements a day. They will be thick, gelatinous, and often very dark. Feeling bloated is normal. Abdominal pain is not normal. If you are constipated, increase the laxative and/or water intake.

2. Gallbladder/Liver Flush

Materials: Olive oil (cold pressed organic), Apple juice (unpasteurized from health food store), Epsom salts or gallbladder formula (J Stones Away), Organic fruit, Whipping cream, Organic coffee, Lemon juice

The liver is the chief organ of metabolism and detoxification. It is vital that it functions optimally. With the onslaught of environmental toxins that we are exposed to today from the air, water, processed foods, and drugs, it is safe to say that we all have a need for liver detoxification. In order for the liver to function properly, it must be free of debris. This procedure aids your body in eliminating the debris. This flush is a simple and natural procedure that helps maintain free-flowing bile and assists the body in eliminating any accumulated matter (stones or sludge composed of stagnate bile or toxins). In all cases, use only reverse osmosis or distilled water.[59]

Mechanism of Action

- In order to remove the sludge or hardened bile and break down the "glue" holding the toxins together, natural forms of acids (malic acid in the apple juice) are employed to allow the gallbladder to readily expel the debris.
- The magnesium (from the Epsom salts) will relax the smooth muscle of the gallbladder wall and bile duct.
- The olive oil causes the gallbladder to contract, forcing the bile sludge and stones out of the gallbladder into the relaxed duct.
- Coffee enemas stimulate the liver to release more bile, flushing the liver and gallbladder.

Procedure

- Drink lots of apple juice for five days.
- On the fifth day, two hours after lunch, dissolve 2 tablespoons of Epsom salts in 30 ounces of warm water and drink it.
- Four hours after lunch, it is best if you do a coffee enema with ¼ cup of Epsom salts in it. Put one cup of brewed organic coffee in an enema bag filled with warm water. The water should be filtered, not directly from the tap. Detailed coffee enema directions are on page 78.
- Six to seven hours after lunch eat fruit with whipped cream on it.
- At bedtime, blend and drink ½ cup of olive oil mixed with lemon juice

(approximately 2 tablespoons).

- Immediately after drinking the oil go to bed and lie on your right side with your knee drawn up to your chest. This helps move the oil from the stomach.
- In the morning, do another coffee enema as above. Drink 3 ounces of water with 1 tablespoon Epsom salts and resume your normal diet.

The morning after the flush, you will find lime-green particles that will float in your bowel movement. This will be the contents of the gallbladder.

3. Tissue/cellular Cleanse
   Materials: Epsom salt, Water, Alkaline punch, Potassium broth, Sea salt, Organic carrot juice

Toxins present in the body from the normal processes of metabolism and environmental sources tend to create a systemic (whole body) acid pH. This tissue/cellular cleanse moves the system into more of an alkaline state to assist in the eliminating of the toxins.

Water plays an important role in our overall health. We simply cannot have health without it, as it plays a vital role in the maintenance of osmotic pressure to carry waste out of our systems. Water transports dead cells and metabolic debris to capillaries, which then transport them to the lymphatic system, then to the bloodstream and then to the kidneys, which eliminate them. In all cases, use only reverse osmosis or distilled water.

Consistently sipping 4 ounces of water every half hour provides the proper amount of water for this process. The human body needs consistent and frequent exposure to water to accomplish detoxification and rebuilding.[60]

Alkaline Punch: Mix the juices of 6 grapefruits, 6 lemons, and 12 oranges in a gallon container, and, if necessary, fill the rest of the container with water.

Potassium Broth: Put one quart of pure water in a pot, bring to a boil, and the peelings (outer ¼") of three organic potatoes. Simmer for 15-30 minutes.

Day One

- Eat as little as necessary of fruits and vegetables only. Do not take any supplements.
- First thing in the morning take 1 tablespoon of Epsom salt dissolved in 3 ounces of warm water.
- Thirty minutes later, repeat
- Thirty minutes later, repeat
- Two hours later, drink 8 ounces of the alkaline punch
- Thirty minutes later, drink four swallows of the alkaline punch
- Thirty minutes later and every thirty minutes, thereafter for the next five hours, drink four swallows of the alkaline punch.

Day Two

- Eat as little as necessary: fruits and vegetables only. Do not take any supplements.
- Drink 4 ounces of water every thirty minutes for an 8-hour period.
- Drink as much fresh carrot juice and potassium broth as you like. Season your broth with sea salt.
- Rest, get some natural sunshine and do some mild exercise.

Day Three

- Resume a normal diet and supplement program.

Coffee Enema

Coffee enemas are widely used by alternative medicine in the treatment of cancer.[61] It is recommended to use them on a regular and ongoing basis. As with the other cleanses, it will affectively remove toxins and cellular waste.

I suggest you shop online for your enema supplies. You may find it difficult to find your supplies, even at a local, medical supply store. There are many different types and prices of enema bags. I purchased a simple, inexpensive bag and found it to be suitable. Please note that the enema tip on the end of the regular hose is not adequate to give a "high enema." This means you will need to buy a special colon tube (DAVOL) size 24 French or 26 French or 28 French. Place this tube on the opposite end of the plastic tube from the enema bag. This colon tube is a soft flexible rubber-like tube around 30 inches in length. It follows the curves of the colon. The colon tube is usually inserted only about 12 to 20 inches into the rectum.

Coffee Enema Directions

1. Just before bedtime each day, make a pot of "drip method" coffee (1 quart). Use only regular, organic coffee made with reverse osmosis or distilled water.
2. Take your coffee enema at the beginning of each day. This will help with any concerns you may have with caffeine intake. If a coffee enema causes a jittery or shaky reaction, the coffee is too strong. The amount of coffee can be adjusted, from 1 teaspoon to 4 tablespoons per quart of water.
3. In the morning, attempt a normal bowel movement. Keep in mine, the raw diet and juicing part of your cancer protocol will greatly help with regular bowel movements. I have found it helpful to first take an enema using reverse osmosis water before attempting the coffee enema. Although this is not necessary, it will clear the bowels, making it easier for you to hold the coffee enema for the required 15 minutes. If you do

this, you do not need to hold the water for a specified time period.

4. Make sure you have assembled your enema bag. The enema bag should not be over 36 inches higher than the rectum. If it is placed too high, the coffee runs into the colon too fast and under too much pressure, causing discomfort. Place one quart of coffee in your enema bag. Allow the coffee to flow to the end of the colon tube, thus eliminating any air in the tube.
5. There are several positions that can be used while inserting the colon tube. Squatting is one. There is also the knee-chest method, with chest and knees on the floor and buttocks in the highest position possible. I found it easiest to lie on my left side until the solution is out of the bag.
6. The colon tube should be lubricated with Vitamin E cream, organic olive oil or an other lubricant that doesn't contain additives or chemicals. Next, slowly insert the tube 12 to 20 inches into the rectum, being careful to use a rotating motion to keep the tube from bending inside the colon.
7. If you are not able to insert the tube past 12 inches, you may have a turn or bend in your colon. Try letting a little of the solution flow into the colon as the tube is being inserted to get past the turn. You can also try taking the tube out a little and then push it back in to get past the turn. If this does not help, then insert the tube only as far as it will go to allow the flow of the liquid. Never force the tube, this could be dangerous.
8. Allow the coffee to begin to flow into the colon. You will need to relax and concentrate on holding the coffee as it flows. Resist the temptation to eliminate your bowels. Once the coffee is completely in, you can remove the tube. Now, time yourself in the following positions: 5 minutes on your left side, 5 minutes on your back, and 5 minutes on your right side. The goal is to hold the coffee enema for 15 minutes. Some people can only retain about 2 cups at a time. If this is the case, take 2 enemas, one right after the other. The coffee may be expelled after the 15 minutes.

◆ Supporting Details

Alternative protocols are very serious medicine. All of the steps working together are powerful, killing cancer cells throughout the body. As a result, there are many dead cells that must be processed out of the body. The colon, liver, gallbladder and lymph system are critical in removing this waste. They must be healthy and free from toxins in order to do this important task. However, for most people, these organs are already burdened with toxins due to years of unhealthy diets and exposure to pollutants. Therefore, it is critical to detox the body, allowing the healing process to continue.

The colon, liver, and gallbladder require detoxification during the treatment process. If this does not occur, a person will run the risk of becoming very ill from the back up of toxins in their body. Since healing is the goal, detoxification is a priority. Detoxification will also open up the lymph system, allowing further removal of toxins.[62]

Laetrile or Vitamin B17

◆ Goal

Take a 500 mg tablet of laetrile as part of your daily regimen.

◆ Supporting Details

Laetrile is derived from the seeds of apricots; it is associated with reducing leukemia and other forms of cancer.[63] It is a natural substance that selectively targets and kills cancer cells safely. It is also found in apple seeds. You will need to purchase vitamin B17 or Laetrile through an online source. It is also easy to buy apricot seeds online. Using both will give you the high, concentrated dose, in combination with nutrients naturally found in the seeds.

It is recommended that a cancer patient take 500 mg of laetrile each day. Take the tablet ½ hour after a meal. If you choose to eat the apricot seeds, begin with 3 to 4 a day and build up to 24 to 40 seeds.[64]

Please Note: B-17 is effective only when taken with the nutrients listed below. If you choose a multi-vitamin, compare the ingredients and be sure to add any supplements to make up any deficiency.[65]

1. Zinc (which is the transport mechanism for laetrile)
2. Vitamin C (build up to 6 grams a day)
3. Manganese
4. Magnesium
5. Selenium
6. Vitamins B6, B9, B12, B15
7. Vitamin A
8. Vitamin E (at least 2,000 I.U.)
9. Iodine
10. Digestive enzymes with pancreatin 10X

Sunshine and Exercise

Two of the best things a person can do for their health are absolutely free. First, exposure to the sun produces Vitamin D. Researchers are convinced that Vitamin D promotes proper function of the heart, bones, brain, and immune system. This vitamin also helps defend against viral infections and has the capability to stifle other infections. More than a century ago, doctors successfully treated tuberculosis patients using sun exposure. Of course, the most exciting news is the connection between Vitamin D levels and cancer risks. For example, it regulates tumor-suppressing proteins and triggers other mechanisms to stop cell growth. In addition, this vitamin limits the process whereby a tumor constructs a netting of blood vessels to feed itself. Michael Holick, a biochemist and endocrinologist at Boston University, sites numerous studies where prostate and ovarian cancer is lower in populations with high sun exposure. Furthermore, he believes that Vitamin D has the greatest impact on colon and breast cancer.[66] In light of this, it is advisable to use plenty of sunscreen protection while enjoying the great outdoors. Second, regular exercise helps a person to feel better, have more energy and perhaps live longer. Most people are aware that it burns calories, but it also combats health conditions and diseases. Regular exercise supports the immune system and can prevent a wide range of health problems, including stroke, type 2 diabetes, arthritis, and certain types of cancer.[67] It is necessary to be sensible and consult a physician when choosing an exercise program. Usually, a person will receive health benefits from just 30 minutes a day. Some of the best forms of exercise are simply bike riding or taking a brisk walk. The important thing is to remain physically active to promote the body's natural ability to heal and remain healthy.

Secondary Protocols and Treatments

Research will help you zero in on all of the possible ways to approach fighting your specific type of cancer. Time and again, I uncovered information, through extensive reading, that helped me make effective decisions. One of the things I discovered was the need to use secondary protocols. These protocols take on a supporting role in your overall efforts. Using additional protocols is like having more weapons in your arsenal against cancer.

Below is a list of some secondary protocols and treatments you can add to the main alternative treatment plan. It is advisable to select at least two secondary treatments to "supercharge" the main protocol. However, there are no limits as to how many treatments you can use. The only thing you must remember is to check the compatibility of your treatments. Again, it is important to do your research. Protocols are well-documented and the research will let you know if certain foods or supplements should not be taken together. With this said, all of the treatments below are excellent ways to aid your body's ability to heal.

Oleander

◆ **Goal**

Take one Rose Laurel OPC Plus® supplement daily.

◆ **Supporting Details**

The oleander plant is toxic to humans in high doses. However, in low doses, it is safe for humans but toxic to cancer cells. Oleander is available as a supplement called Rose Laurel OPC Plus®. This supplement has been widely used by both cancer and aids patients, so the dose and safety is well established. It is more than 90% effective against many types of cancer, including late stage cancer.[68] This supplement can be purchased online at Utopia Silver Supplements.

Baking Soda and Maple Syrup

◆ **Goal**

Take one to three servings of the baking soda and maple syrup mixture daily.

Purchase 100 % organic maple syrup (grade B) and aluminum-free baking soda. Measure 1 level teaspoon baking soda to 3 level teaspoons maple syrup. Stir the mixture over low heat for 5 to 10 minutes. Be careful not to burn the mixture. Keep it just warm enough so that it does not burn. The two ingredients will combine for a pleasant taste. Always make it fresh.[69]

◆ **Supporting Details**

The maple syrup targets cancer cells because the cells consume glucose.

As a cancer cell takes in the maple syrup, it also brings in the baking soda. The baking soda is very alkaline. This protocol works by killing the microbes inside the cancer cell.

Asparagus

(Not recommended for anyone on blood thinners)

◆ Goal

Eat 8 tablespoons of asparagus daily.

1. Cook the organic asparagus
2. Puree the cooked asparagus
3. Eat four tablespoons, twice a day

◆ Supporting Details

Asparagus is an excellent cancer-fighting vegetable. It is a valuable source of glutathione, a detoxifying compound. Also, asparagus is packed with antioxidants, giving it the ability to neutralize cell-damaging free radicals. It is part of the original list of cruciferous vegetables in the main protocol of the raw food diet. This protocol is very simple and inexpensive.[70]

Wheatgrass

◆ Goal

Juice 1 to 2 ounces of wheatgrass five days a week. Drink half of the juice immediately and the other half of the juice four hours later.

◆ Supporting Details

One of the goals for killing cancer cells is to get oxygen back into the cells. Wheatgrass contains chlorophyll, and this increases hemoglobin production, allowing for more oxygen to get into the cells. Wheatgrass also contains at least 13 vitamins, many minerals and trace elements. It also contains enzymes, laetrile and other nutrients. The best reason for juicing wheatgrass may be the oxygen availability that the chlorophyll provides.[71]

Essiac Tea

The essiac formula was originally used by Indians and discovered by a Canadian nurse named Rene Caisse to treat terminally-ill cancer patients. Her story is remarkable in that she believed in the healing power of these herbs and put her convictions into action treating terminally-ill patients. The following list is the basic ingredients of the tea formula.[72] You also have the option of purchasing essiac tea online.

◆ Goal

Mix 2 ounces essiac tea with 2 ounces pure water, boil and sip. Drink 3 times daily ½ hour before eating or 2 hours after eating, preferably after arising, in the afternoon and before retiring.

Essiac consists of four herbs: 6 ½ cups of burdock root, 1 lb. of sheep sorrel, ¼ lb. of slipper elm bark and 1 ounce of Turkish rhubarb root.

Boil 1 cup of herb mix in 2 gallons pure water for 10 minutes, let sit 6 hours, stir, let sit 6 more hours, stir, reboil, strain, and bottle in sterile amber glass bottles. Store in a dark place. Refrigerate after opening.

Resource for ingredients:
Herb Products Co: 11012 Magnolia Blvd., North Hollywood, CA, 91601
Phone: 818-761-0351, Website: www.herbproducts.com

◆ Supporting Details

The herbs possess antioxidant and anti-cancer properties, according to research conducted at the European Institute of Oncology. The findings were reported in the March 2006 issue of the Journal of Ethnopharmacology. Researchers claim that the four herbs demonstrated natural protection against cancer. The tea may also be beneficial in treating breast cancer according to a report in the 2007 edition of the journal Anticancer Research.[73]

TEST AND SCREENING

Orthodox medicine primarily uses CT scans, mammograms, bone scans, and MRI's to diagnosis and to assess the condition of a cancer patient. These types of imaging capabilities provide a picture of where the cancer is in the patient's body. While these may be valuable tools for the oncologist, they are not in the best interest of the patient.

Today, there are serious health implications from exposure to radiation through diagnostic scans. Some physicians are raising concerns about the safety of such procedures — most notably, an increase in cancer risk. A single CT scan packs a mega-dose of radiation — as much as 750 times that of a conventional chest X-ray.[74] It really is something to think about when looking at the possible accumulation of exposure for a cancer patient in need of long-term treatment assessment.

This adverse information led me to an alternative screening process. I found an ideal option at the Navarro Medical Clinic. This clinic offers human chorionic gonadotrophin (HCG) immunoassay urinalysis testing.[75] This is a non-invasive, accurate screening test for cancer. It determines how actively the body is producing unnecessary cells or controlling cell production at a normal level. This test provides a cancer patient with a cost-effective way to track the success of his/her treatment and check the status of remission. Details about this test can be found at: www.navarromedicalclinic.com

PART FOUR

MY MEAL PLAN

A raw food diet is an essential part of your treatment plan. With this comes the challenge of selecting the right foods for each meal, as well as avoiding those that are not recommended. At first, you may feel limited, but in truth, your meals will be as varied as your creativity. In this section, you will find a list of foods to plan your meals around and menu ideas, which include many of these different foods. The menus will serve as a guideline for making your meals both nutritious and delicious.

◆ FOODS FOR MEAL PLANNING

1. Leafy Greens

   Spinach is a favorite leafy green, but other good ones include kale, bok choi, collards, dark-green romaine (skip iceberg), and other similar greens. Try to build several of your meals around these greens, as they are high in fiber, vitamins and minerals.

2. Avocados

   These are a source of good fats and good flavor. Avocados are great in salads, sandwiches, wraps and more.

3. Tomatoes

   Add these to flavor any dish — salads, sandwiches, pastas, soups, anything.

4. Fruits

   Fruits are filled with fiber and vitamins but are low in calories. The best selection includes green apples, grapes, blueberries, strawberries, blackberries, pineapple, and plums. Dark color fruits are best. They are good as a snack, juiced, chopped up, or as a side dish. Use fruits to complete any of your three main meals. You can add them to cereal, like oatmeal, for breakfast.

5. Nuts
   They are full of fiber and good fats and protein. Choose almonds, walnuts or pecans over peanuts. You can chop them up and put them in hot cereal, salads, stir fries, or just eat them as snacks. Try almond butter or sunflower-seed butter on toast.

6. Beans
   Beans are a great source of fiber and protein, low in calories. You can eat beans all day long. I like them in chili, soups, tacos and more. Get a variety — red, black, pinto, white, and lentils.

7. Whole grains
   This is a broad category that includes all kinds of hot and cold cereals, breads, wraps, brown rice and more. Select sprouted grains, English muffins or cereals. Absolutely no "wheat flour" or "enriched wheat flour." It is simply not nutritious.

8. Olive oil
   You need fats, but they must be the good kind. I recommend olive oil, in addition to the flaxseed oil used in this treatment plan. Again, nuts and avocados also provide good fats.

9. Lean protein. On this "raw" diet, you are receiving vegetable protein — lots of greens, beans and nuts. Whole grains also contain protein, as do other vegetables. It is not hard to meet your daily requirements, even if exercise increases your requirements.

10. Lean calcium. Rice and almond milk are a good source of calcium.

◆ MENU IDEAS

This information is purposely presented in a simple format. It is meant to give you a starting point for making good decisions, within the guidelines of the raw food diet plan. I included meal ideas that have worked well for me. Using these simple ideas, you should be able to create your own daily meal plans.

I believe these foods are all good choices. However, it is important that you balance your diet. Make sure you alternate menu options and keep the ingredients varied. This will ensure you receive a proper intake of vitamins and minerals. Simply choose one of the meals from each category, each day, and enjoy up to three snacks per day.

Breakfast

1. Organic hot or cold cereal with rice milk (Top with berries, nuts, or flaxseed)
2. Sprouted-grain toast with sunflower seed or other nut butter
3. Fruit on the side
4. Fried brown rice — fry up with olive oil, onions, mushrooms, and green vegetables

Lunch

1. Sprouted bread sandwich or wrap. Any combination of vegetables. Try tomatoes, spinach or other greens, avocados, hummus, bell peppers with organic dijon mustard, pesto and/or olive oil.
2. Organic pita bread with hummus. Add olives, tomatoes, peppers, raw spinach and sprouts.
3. Vegetable burger on a sprouted-grain bun top with lots of vegetables (greens, sprouts, tomatoes and avocados). Use a recipe that does not

include eggs or soy; soy is not recommended. Organic sweet potato fries (use olive oil and a little sea salt)

4. Salads using spinach or other greens, tomatoes, avocados, feta cheese, nuts, and maybe some chopped fruit or berries. Dress with organic olive oil and vinegar.
5. Snacks. Cut organic carrots, broccoli, cauliflower, or edamame dipped in organic hummus.
6. Almonds, walnuts, or pecans
7. Protein shake made with vegetable protein, along with rice milk, frozen berries, bananas and ground flaxseed.
8. Fruits

Dinner

1. Vegetable stir-fry. Stir-fry some onions and chopped vegetables — various greens such as kale, bok choi and swiss chard work well. You can also add broccoli, bell peppers, tomatoes, mushrooms and carrots, as well as sliced nuts. Season with black pepper, garlic, sea salt and ginger. This is great served over brown rice.
2. Tacos. Some low-fat refried beans and/or black beans on soft organic corn tortillas with organic salsa, greens, tomatoes, and corn.
3. Vegetarian chili with brown rice or sprouted-grain bread and olive oil.
4. Brown rice spaghetti or other brown rice pasta. Cook some onions, tomatoes and bell peppers with tomato sauce and basil. Add some fresh Parmesan over an organic pasta sauce.
5. Soup. Choose a favorite recipe for homemade organic soup.

PART FIVE

MY JUICING RECIPES

The recipes provided in this section include a variety of vegetables and fruits important for nutrition and healing. As always, only use fresh, organic produce. Be careful to wash and remove seeds from fruits and vegetables before juicing. Also, remember to drink the juice right away to keep nutrient loss at a minimum. These recipes are simple and easy to make. Feel free to combine favorite vegetables and fruits into your own juicing recipes. Enjoy!

◆ VEGETABLE JUICES

1. Cabbage: 1 Cup Red Cabbage, 1 Beet, 2 Carrots, ½ of a Sweet Red Pepper, 1 Orange, 1 Green Apple and 1″ of Ginger
2. Kale: 1 Bunch of Kale, 4 Carrots, ½ of a Cucumber, 2 Stalks of Celery, 1 Green Apple, 1 Lemon, ¼" of Ginger and 1 Beet (greens and bulb)
3. Broccoli: 1 Broccoli Spear, 2 Apples and 4 Carrots
4. Cucumber: 1 Cucumber, 2 Stalks of Celery, 1 Apple, ½ Lemon, ½″ of Ginger, ½ of a Green Chard Leaf, Cilantro, 3-5 Kale Leaves and 1 Cup Spinach
5. Cauliflower: ½ of a Head of Cauliflower, 1 Handful of Spinach, 2 Large Red Delicious Apples and ½ of a Lime (peeled)
6. Spinach: 1 Handful of Spinach, 4 Carrots and 2 Green Apples
7. Sweet Potato: 1 Sweet Potato, 1″ of Ginger, 3 Red Delicious Apples and 2 Stalks of Celery

8. Swiss Chard: 4 Leaves of Swiss Chard, 4 Carrots, ½ of a Cucumber and 4 Apples
9. Wheatgrass: 2-3" Round of Wheatgrass, 4 Carrots, ½ of a Beetroot, 3 Stalks of Celery and 1 Large Apple

◆ FRUIT JUICES

1. Pineapple: ¼ of a Pineapple, 1 Cup Blueberries and ¼" of Ginger
2. Berries: 2 Cups of Strawberries, 2 Cups of Blueberries and 1½ Cups of Raspberries
3. Cherries: 1 Pint of Cherries, 2 Apples, and 1 Orange (peel the skin)
4. Cranberries: 1 Handful of Cranberries and 2-3 Apples
5. Grapes: 15 Grapes, 1 Orange (peel the skin) and 4 Carrots
6. Papaya: 1 Medium Size Papaya and 5 Strawberries
7. Pear: 1 Pear, 1 Apple and 10 Grapes
8. Pomegranate: 1 Pomegranate (de-seeded) only juice the seeds discard rind and membranes and 2 Apples

PART SIX

MY FINAL THOUGHTS

Every thought in this book was carefully chosen with the singular purpose of providing both spiritual and practical guidance in helping a cancer patient find their path to healing. For me, there is no separating the spiritual from the medical side of healing. I have experienced first hand the love and compassion of the "Great Physician." When no one could calm my fears, I heard His voice whisper words of assurance to my troubled soul. He changed the measure of my life and the dimension of my faith. There are no limits to my God and the love He has for me. He traveled with me through the pages of my Bible, showing me a treasure room of promises.

For the eyes of the LORD run to and fro throughout the whole earth, to shew himself strong in the behalf of them whose heart is perfect toward him... II Chronicles 16:9

From His Word, I learned to let God be strong on my behalf. I surrendered to Him the things I could not change, and in turn, He gave me strength for every situation. He showed me that praying was as necessary as breathing. In every moment there was an opportunity to feel His presence and to rise above my circumstances. In truth, He became the source of my healing in every possible way.

There is no one in my life that has not been affected in some way by my experience. Certainly, my family has been transformed during the past two years. My children know they are witnesses to a miracle. They speak often about the early days surrounding my diagnosis and the realization of God's power to heal a life-threatening illness. Individually, they have gained a level of faith not possible without the knowledge of God answering their prayers. Together, Manny and I have seen God completely change the course of our lives. Following God's leading, Manny made the decision to end his sixteen-year career in the medical industry in favor of a full-time position at our church. He is now ministering as the principal of Stockton Christian Academy and as a pastor on staff at Christian Life Center. We both agree that God used our collective experiences to usher us into a time of believing and serving Him for greater things.

God has orchestrated every detail of my life. Although, God could have healed me instantly, I believe He intended my experience to result in helping others through the writing of this book. I am grateful for His guidance in leading me to the answers within these pages. The lessons I learned were valuable both to my soul and to the healing of my body. It is my desire that everyone reading this book will find the courage to partner with God for their healing.

PART SEVEN

My Spiritual Strength

During my illness, the Bible was my daily prescription for strength and comfort. Nothing could replace what God did for me through the reading of His Word. I have listed here many of the Scriptures that I used to build my faith. I hope you will be encouraged to rely on God's promises and to allow Him to speak to you through His very own words.

◆ Healing

1. *But he was wounded for our transgressions, he was bruised for our iniquities: the chastisement of our peace was upon him; and with his stripes we are healed.* Isaiah 53:5

2. *Is any sick among you? let him call for the elders of the church; and let them pray over him, anointing him with oil in the name of the Lord: And the prayer of faith shall save the sick, and the Lord shall raise him up; and if he have committed sins, they shall be forgiven him. Confess your faults one to another, and pray one for another, that ye may be healed. The effectual fervent prayer of a righteous man availeth much.* James 5:14-16

3. *And one of them, when he saw that he was healed, turned back, and with a loud voice glorified God,* Luke 17:15

4. *O LORD my God, I cried unto thee, and thou hast healed me.* Psalm 30:2

5. *Heal me, O LORD, and I shall be healed; save me, and I shall be saved: for thou art my praise.* Jeremiah 17:14

6. *Then they cry unto the LORD in their trouble, and he saveth them out of their distresses. He sent his word, and healed them, and delivered them from their destructions. Oh that men would praise the LORD for his goodness, and for his wonderful works to the children of men!* Psalm 107:19-21
7. *They shall take up serpents; and if they drink any deadly thing, it shall not hurt them; they shall lay hands on the sick, and they shall recover.* Mark 16:18
8. *That thy way may be known upon earth, thy saving health among all nations.* Psalm 67:2
9. *Then shall thy light break forth as the morning, and thine health shall spring forth speedily: and thy righteousness shall go before thee; the glory of the LORD shall be thy rereward.* Isaiah 58:8
10. *But unto you that fear my name shall the Sun of righteousness arise with healing in his wings; and ye shall go forth, and grow up as calves of the stall.* Malachi 4:2
11. *Bless the LORD, O my soul, and forget not all his benefits: Who for giveth all thine iniquities; who healeth all thy diseases;* Psalm 103:2,3
12. *And Jesus went forth, and saw a great multitude, and was moved with compassion toward them, and he healed their sick.* Matthew 14:14

◆ Fear

1. *The LORD is my light and my salvation; whom shall I fear? the LORD is the strength of my life; of whom shall I be afraid?* Psalm 27:1
2. *Wait on the LORD: be of good courage, and he shall strengthen thine heart: wait, I say, on the LORD.* Psalm 21:14

3. *Fear thou not; for I am with thee: be not dismayed; for I am thy God: I will strengthen thee; yea, I will help thee; yea, I will uphold thee with the right hand of my righteousness.* Isaiah 41:10
4. *For I the LORD thy God will hold thy right hand, saying unto thee, Fear not; I will help thee.* Isaiah 41:13
5. *For God hath not given us the spirit of fear; but of power, and of love, and of a sound mind.* II Timothy 1:7
6. *So that we may boldly say, The Lord is my helper, and I will not fear what man shall do unto me.* Hebrews 13:6
7. *And the LORD, he it is that doth go before thee; he will be with thee, he will not fail thee, neither forsake thee: fear not, neither be dismayed.* Deuteronomy 31:8
8. *There is no fear in love; but perfect love casteth out fear: because fear hath torment. He that feareth is not made perfect in love.* I John 4:18
9. *Yea, though I walk through the valley of the shadow of death, I will fear no evil: for thou art with me; thy rod and thy staff they comfort me.* Psalm 23:4
10. *Peace I leave with you, my peace I give unto you: not as the world giveth, give I unto you. Let not your heart be troubled, neither let it be afraid.* John 14:27

◆ FAITH

1. *But let all those that put their trust in thee rejoice: let them ever shout for joy, because thou defendest them: let them also that love thy name be joyful in thee.* Psalm 5:11
2. *Hear my prayer, O LORD, give ear to my supplications: in thy faithfulness answer me, and in thy righteousness.* Psalm 143:1

3. *And they that know thy name will put their trust in thee: for thou, LORD, hast not forsaken them that seek thee.* Psalm 9:10
4. *He that dwelleth in the secret place of the most High shall abide under the shadow of the Almighty. I will say of the LORD, He is my refuge and my fortress: my God; in him will I trust.* Psalm 91:1,2
5. *Some trust in chariots, and some in horses: but we will remember the name of the LORD our God.* Psalm 20:7
6. *God is our refuge and strength, a very present help in trouble.* Psalm 46:1
7. *The LORD is my rock, and my fortress, and my deliverer; my God, my strength, in whom I will trust; my buckler, and the horn of my salvation, and my high tower.* Psalm 18:2
8. *Know therefore that the LORD thy God, he is God, the faithful God, which keepeth covenant and mercy with them that love him and keep his commandments to a thousand generations;* Deuteronomy 7:9
9. *Hast thou not known? hast thou not heard, that the everlasting God, the LORD, the Creator of the ends of the earth, fainteth not, neither is weary? there is no searching of his understanding.* Isaiah 40:28
10. *Being confident of this very thing, that he which hath begun a good work in you will perform it until the day of Jesus Christ:* Philippians 1:6
11. *Let us therefore come boldly unto the throne of grace, that we may obtain mercy, and find grace to help in time of need.* Hebrews 4:16
12. *Therefore I say unto you, What things soever ye desire, when ye pray, believe that ye receive them, and ye shall have them.* Mark 11:24
13. *And this is the confidence that we have in him, that, if we ask any thing according to his will, he heareth us: And if we know that he hear us, whatsoever we ask, we know that we have the petitions that we desired of him.* I John 5:14,15

14. *For we walk by faith, not by sight:* II Corinthians 5:7
15. *And all things, whatsoever ye shall ask in prayer, believing, ye shall receive.* Matthew 21:22
16. *If ye abide in me, and my words abide in you, ye shall ask what ye will, and it shall be done unto you.* John 15:7
17. *Jesus Christ the same yesterday, and to day, and for ever.* Hebrews 13:8
18. *Thou wilt keep him in perfect peace, whose mind is stayed on thee: because he trusteth in thee.* Isaiah 26:3
19. *Now faith is the substance of things hoped for, the evidence of things not seen.* Hebrews 11:1
20. *And whatsoever ye shall ask in my name, that will I do, that the Father may be glorified in the Son. If ye shall ask any thing in my name, I will do it.* John 14:13,14
21. *So then faith cometh by hearing, and hearing by the word of God.* Romans 10:17
22. *Again I say unto you, That if two of you shall agree on earth as touching any thing that they shall ask, it shall be done for them of my Father which is in heaven.* Matthew 18:19
23. *For the eyes of the LORD run to and fro throughout the whole earth, to shew himself strong in the behalf of them whose heart is perfect toward him...* II Chronicles 16:9

Scripture Key Rings

My experience has proven to me the value of keeping the Word of God at hand. As I mentioned earlier in this book, I created individual Scripture cards and placed them on a key ring. This allowed me to easily tuck them into to a handbag, a pocket or a briefcase. In this formate, they were available whenever I needed encouragement or a reminder of God's promises.

This same Scripture key ring, Fight of Faith, is available through the Women's Ministries at Christian Life Center. In addition, there are five other topics to choose from with twelve Bible verses on each key ring. They are beautifully designed using bright colors and laminated for safekeeping. If you are interested in purchasing any of the Scripture key rings, please use the information provided below. All proceeds benefit the Women's Ministries at Christian Life Center.

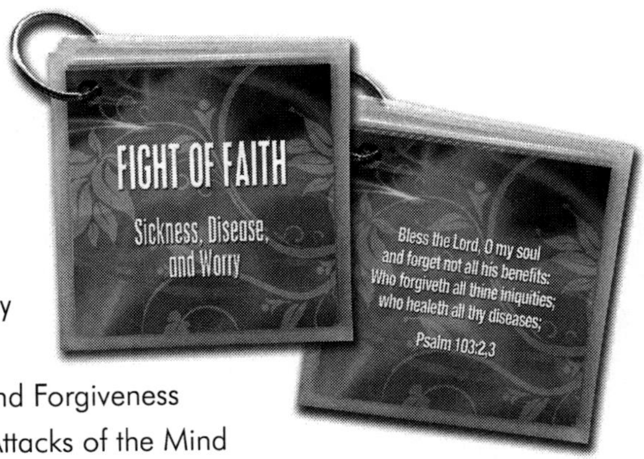

◆ Topics

1. Fight of Faith
2. Pride and Jealousy
3. Spiritual Attacks
4. Bitterness, Hurt and Forgiveness
5. Depression and Attacks of the Mind
6. Fear of Rejection, Fear of Worth and Insecurity Through Fornication

◆ Ordering Information

Scripture Key Rings are $5 each. *(This does not include shipping.)*
CHRISTIAN LIFE CENTER
209-957-4027
Please visit our store at www.clministry.com

PART EIGHT

My Resources

There are hundreds of websites, books, magazines and films that provide information about alternative medicine. These resources will equip you to make positive decisions about your health. Below are just a few of the resources available for research and for purchasing health related products.

◆ Websites

1. Cancer Tutor. This is a comprehensive research website for cancer. www.cancertutor.com
2. Dr. Lorraine Day. Dr. Day speaks frankly about her experience healing her own cancer safely and naturally. www.drday.com
3. Gerson Institute. The Gerson Institute is dedicated to curing cancer and other so called "incurable" diseases. www.gerson.org
4. Dr. William Kelley. Dr. Kelley provides a testimonial video and detailed information about alternative treatment for cancer. www.drkelley.com
5. World Without Cancer. This site has a wealth of information on cancer treatment using vitamin B17 therapy. www.worldwithoutcancer.org
6. Oasis of Hope Hospital. This hospital is located in Tijuana, Mexico. It offers alternative cancer treatment. www.oasisofhope.com
7. Cyto Pharma de Mexico, S.A. This site offers vitamin B17 products. www.cytopharmaonline.com

8. Independent Cancer Research Foundation, Inc. This is a good resource for alternative treatments. www.new-cancer-treatments.org
9. Cancer-Free. Bill Henderson offers alternative treatment information and coaching for cancer patients. www.beating-cancer-gently.com
10. The Consumer Lab. Here you will find detailed reviews and research on vitamin and mineral products. www.consumerlab.com
11. Vitacost. This site offers health products. Vitacost is a good source for most of the items mentioned in this book. www.vitacost.com
12. Free Drinking Water. On this site you will find product information on reverse osmosis water filtration systems. www.freedrinkingwater.com

◆ BOOKS

1. *Gerson, Max M.D.. A Cancer Therapy. New York: Kensington Publishing Corp, 1958, 6th Edition.*
2. *Kelley, William D. One Answer To Cancer. Mokelumne Hill, 1994.*
3. *Henderson, Bill. Cancer-Free. Booklocker, 2011, 4th Edition.*
4. *Budwig, Johanna MD. Cancer The Problem and The Solution. Nexus Gmbh, 2008, 1st Edition.*
5. *Moss, Ralph MD. Questioning Chemotherapy. Equinox, 1995.*
6. *Brownstein, David MD. Iodine, Why You Need It, Why You Can't Live Without It. Medical Alternatives Press, 2009, 4th Edition.*
7. *Richardson, John A. MD. Laetrile Case Histories. California: American Media, 2005, 5th Edition.*
8. *Griffin, G. Edward. World Without Cancer: The Story of Vitamin B17. California: American Media, 2003, 17th Edition.*

9. *Matthias, Rath MD. Cellular Health Series: Cancer. Santa Clara: MR Publishing, Inc., 2002, 1st Edition.*

10. *Colbert, Don MD. The Seven Pillars of Health. Florida: Siloam, 2007, 1st Edition.*

11. *Heinerman, John. Heinerman's New Encyclopedia of Fruits & Vegetables. New York: Parker Publishing Company Inc., 1995.*

◆ CD's

1. *Cancer Doesn't Scare Me Anymore* - Dr. Lorraine Day, MD
2. *You Can't Improve on God* - Dr. Lorraine Day, MD
3. *Systemic Enzyme Therapy* - Dr. William Wong ND, PhD
4. *Your Road to Health* - Michael V. Rentas

◆ Films

1. *The Gerson Miracle*. This video covers the history of natural treatment for cancer at the Gerson Institute. It can be purchased online at Walmart or Best Buy. Also it is available to view on Netflix.
2. *Healing Cancer.* A film that questions traditional medicine and offers natural alternatives for healing the body. It is available on Netflix.
3. *The Beautiful Truth*. This is a documentary investigating the premise that diet can cure cancer and other diseases. It is available on Netflix.
4. *Dying To Have Known*. This film is about a holistic cancer treatment dismissed by the American medical establishment. It is available on Netflix.
5. *Food Matters*. A documentary that explores the failure of traditional medicine to treat and cure disease. It focuses on nutrition as a cure for disease. It is available on Netflix.

NOTES

1. "Big Pharma Spends More on Advertising Than Research and Development, Study Finds," Science Daily, http://www.sciencedaily.com/releases/2008/01/080 105140107.htm.

2. "12 Deadly Diseases Cured in the 20th Century," Discovery Health, http://health.howstuffworks.com/diseases-conditions/rare/12-deadly-diseases-cured-in-the-20th-century.htm.

3. "Part 1 of 3: What Causes Cancer at the Systemic Level," Cancer Tutor, http://www.cancertutor.com/Articles/What_Causes_Cancer.html.

4. "Understanding and Managing Chemotherapy Side Effects," Cancer Care, http://www.cancercare.org/publications/24-understanding_and_managing_chemotherapy_side_effects#possible-side-effects

5. "Managing Side Effects," Cancer Treatment Centers of America, http://www.cancercenter.com/after-care-services/managing-side-effects.cfm

6. "Part 1 of 3: What Causes Cancer at the Systemic Level," Cancer Tutor, http://www.cancertutor.com/Articles/What_Causes_Cancer.html

7. "Supplement Strategy - Iodine," Breast Cancer Choices, http://www.breastcancerchoices.org/iodine.html

8. *Don Colbert MD., The Seven Pillars of Health. (Florida: Siloam, 2007), 208.*

9. "Diet Details and Warnings," Cancer Tutor, http://www.cancertutor.com/Articles/What_Causes_Cancer.html

10. "The Benefits of Staying Hydrated," Prevention, http://www.prevention.com/biggest-loser-fitness-drinking-water

11. "The Truth About Our Environment and Water," Free Drinking Water, http://www.freedrinkingwater.com/water-purification-need.htm

12. Ibid.

13. "The Importance of Water and Your Health," Free Drinking Water, http://www.freedrinkingwater.com/water-education/water-health.htm

14. Neal D. Barnard, Patricia Bertron, Suzanne Havala, Jennifer Keller, Gabrielle Turner-McGrievy, Martin Root, Any Joy Lanou, Kristine Kieswer, Brenda Davis, *Healthy Eating For Life to Prevent and Treat Cancer* (New York: John Wiley & Sons, 2002), 92-93.

15. "Diet Details and Warnings," Cancer Tutor, http://www.cancertutor.com/Articles/What_Causes_Cancer.html

16. "Benefits of Sprouted Grains," Natural Therapy Pages, http://www.naturaltherapypages.com.au/article/Benefits_Sprouted_Grains

17. "What are the Benefits of Organic Brown Rice?," Livestrong, http://www.livestrong.com/article/401935-what-are-the-benefits-of-organic-brown-rice/

18. The American Institute for Cancer Research's Program for Cancer Prevention, *Stopping Cancer Before It Starts* (New York: Golden Books, 1999), 178.

19. "Discover the Health Benefits Juicing Carrots," Natural News, http://www.naturalnews.com/034511_carrots_juicing_health_benefits.html

20. "The Benefits of Apple Cider Vinegar," Global Healing Center, http://www.globalhealingcenter.com/natural-health/the-benefits-of-apple-cider-vinegar/

21. "Spirulina – Packed With Protein, B12 and Iron," Natural News, http://www.naturalnews.com/033698_spirulina_superfood.html

22. "Spirulina – Health Benefits of Liquid Chlorophyll," Energise For Life, http://www.energiseforlife.com/wordpress/2009/02/11/health-benefits-of-liquid-chlorophyll/

23. David Servan-Schreiber, MD, PhD, *Anticancer a New Way of Life* (New York: Viking, 2009), 118.

24. "Fruit Juices," Cancer Tutor, http://www.cancertutor.com/Cancer/Raw Food.html

25. "Which Juicer is Right for You," Harvest Essentials, http://www.harvestessentials .com/whatjuicisri.html

26. Ibid.

27. "The Gerson Guide to Juicers," Juicers, http://gerson.org/gerpress/gerson -guide-to-juicers/

28. "Which Juicer is Right for You," Harvest Essentials, http://www.harvestessentials .com/whatjuicisri.html

29. Michael V. Rentas, *Your Road to Health*, Cellect/Budwig and More, 2010, compact disc

30. "What is Aerobic Respiration?,"Wisegeek, http://www.wisegeek.com/what -is-aerobic-respiration.htm

31. Michael V. Rentas, *Your Road to Health*, Cellect/Budwig and More, 2010, compact disc

32. "What is Ionized Water and are There Real Health Benefits From Drinking This Type of Water?," Free Drinking Water, http://www.freedrinkingwater.com/water_health/health2/health-benefits-from-drinking-ionized-water.htm

33. "How to Make the Budwig Diet Mixture," Cancer Tutor, http://www.cancer tutor.com/Other03/Make_Budwig.html

34. "Dr. Johanna Budwig Biography," Budwig Center, http://www.budwigcenter.com/johanna-budwig-biography.php

35. Ibid.

36. Ibid.

37. Ibid.

38. Donald R. Yance, Jr., and Arlene Valentine, *Herbal Medicine, Healing & Cancer* (Chicago: Keats Publishing, 1999), 178.

39. "Why Should I Take a Vitamin for My Health?," NBC News, http://today.msnbc.msn.com/id/9402607/ns/today-today_health/t/why-should-i-take-vitamin-my-health/#.UCRNaBxUNc1

40. "Iodine for Health," Lewrockwell, http://www.lewrockwell.com/miller/miller20.html

41. "Kryolic Moducare Immune Formula," Vitacost, http://www.vitacost.com/kyolic-moducare-180-capsules

42. "Coenzyme A the Master Enzyme," Electronic Healing, http://www.electronichealing.co.uk/products/coenzyme.htm

43. "Vitacost ToCoQ10®," Vitacost, http://www.vitacost.com/vitacost-tocoq10

44. "Spirulina (Arthrospira platensis)," Herbwisdom, http://www.herbwisdom.com/herb-spirulina.html

45. Maureen Kennedy Salaman, *Nutrition: The Cancer Answer II* (Mountain View: Statford Publishing, 1996), 331.

46. "What Are the Benefits of Vitamin B Complex for Stress?," Livestrong, http://www.livestrong.com/article/371982-what-are-the-benefits-of-vitamin-b-complex-for-stress/

47. "Calcium Magnesium Zinc Benefits," Livestrong, http://www.livestrong.com/article/371982-what-are-the-benefits-of-vitamin-b-complex-for-stress/

48. Ibid.

49. "Nature's Way GTF Chromium Polynicotinate," Vitacost, http://www.vitacost.com/natures-way-gtf-chromium-polynicotinate

50. "Branch Chain Amino Acids Benefits," Livestrong, http://www.livestrong.com/article/440616-branch-chain-amino-acid-benefits/

51. "Mega Digestive Enzymes With Pancretin 10X," Vitacost, http://www.vitacost.com/natures-way-gtf-chromium-polynicotinate

52. "Benefits of Vitamin E," Discovery Fit and Health, http://health.howstuffworks.com/wellness/food-nutrition/vitamin-supplements/benefits-of-vitamin-e.htm

53. "Health Benefits of Turmeric – The Best of a Truly Amazing Food," Natural Society, http://naturalsociety.com/overcoming-pharmaceuticals-top-health-benefits-of-turmeric/

54. Michio Kushi and Alex Jack, *The Cancer Prevention Diet* (New York: St. Martin's Press, 2009), 154.

55. "Benefits Of Vitamin A," Discovery Fit and Health, http://health.howstuffworks.com/wellness/food-nutrition/vitamin-supplements/benefits-of-vitamin-a.htm

56. "Health Benefits of Liquid Chlorophyll," Energize for Life, http://www.energiseforlife.com/wordpress/2009/02/11/health-benefits-of-liquid-chlorophyll/

57. "What is a Detoxification Program," Naturally Empowered, http://www.naturallyempowered.com/html/detox.html

58. "Alternative Medicine," Living Waters Medical Spa and Wellness Center, http://www.viglionemd.com/alternativemedicine.html

59. Ibid.

60. Ibid.

61. "The Coffee Enema," One Answer to Cancer, http://www.drkelley.com/CANLIVER55.html#_Toc434239890

62. Ibid

63. Michael Murray, Tim Birdsall, Joseph E. Pizzorno, and Paul Reilly, *How to Prevent and Treat Cancer with Natural Medicine* (New York: Riverhead Books, 2002), 61.

64. "How to Obtain Laetrile or Vitamin B17," Cancer Tutor, http://www.cancertutor.com/Cancer/Laetrile.html

65. "Laetrile/Vitamin B17 Treatment for Cancer," Cancer Tutor, http://www.cancertutor.com/Cancer/Laetrile.html

66. "The Power of D," Science News, http://www.sciencenews.org/view/feature/id/332009/title/The_power_of_D

67. "Fitness," Mayo Clinic, http://www.mayoclinic.com/health/exercise/HQ01676/NSECTIONGROUP=2

68. "Tony Isaacs Oleander Protocol for Cancer and Aids," Cancer Tutor, http:// www.cancertutor.com/Cancer02/Oleander.html

69. "Jim Kelmun Protocol Supplemental Cancer Treatment," Cancer Tutor, http://www.cancertutor.com/Cancer02/Kelmun.html

70. "Inexpensive Yet Potent Cancer Treatments," Cancer Tutor, http://www.cancertutor.com/faq/faq_inexpensive.html

71. "Ann Wigmore Wheatgrass Treatment for Cancer," Cancer Tutor, http://www.cancertutor.com/Cancer/Wheatgrass.html

72. "The Essiac Benefits of Tea," Livestrong, http://www.livestrong.com/article/271727-the-essiac-benefits-of-tea/

73. Ibid.

74. "What About CT Scan Radiation?," Electricsense, http://electricsense.com/1544/what-about-ct-scan-radiation/

75. "HCG Urine Immunoassay," Navarro Medical Clinic Dr. Efren Navarro, MD, http://www.navarromedicalclinic.com/